SMARTER DIETER SECRETS

Unlocking the Secrets of Weight Loss & Reset Your Metabolism

The Complete Guide To Weight Loss, Burn Belly

Fat, And Keep It Off For Good For Woman

With Diet Cookbooks

Susan Firesong

Bonus Resources

Thanks for getting this book

Here are some bonus resources that can help you lose weight and keep it off

1. Get My #1 Recommended Supplement - Exipure

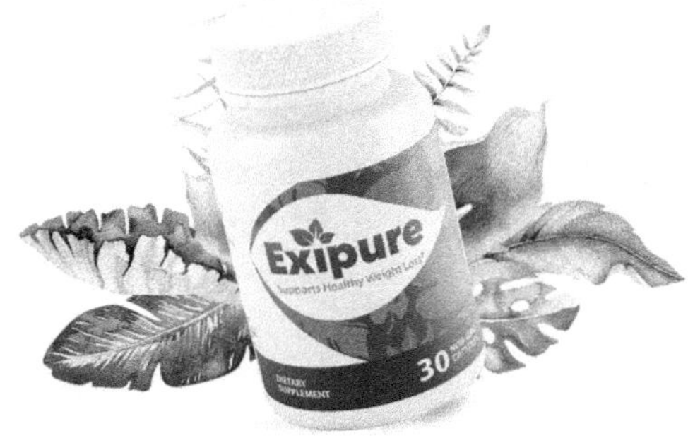

My go-to supplement for healthy weight loss
You can learn more about it and get your discount bottle at
https://smarterdieter.org/exipure/

2. Join my Recommended Workout Program
- Yoga Burn Challenge

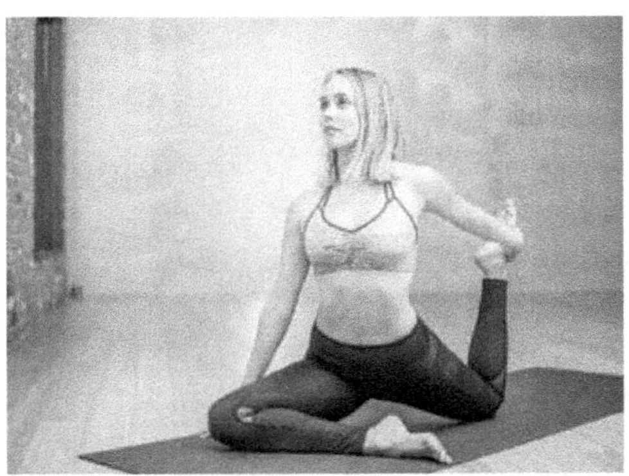

Join the online challenge that will help you lose weight quickly
Sign up now at https://smarterdieter.org/yoga/

TABLE OF CONTENTS

PART 1

THE BLUEPRINT OF WEIGHT LOSS

YES, YOU CAN!

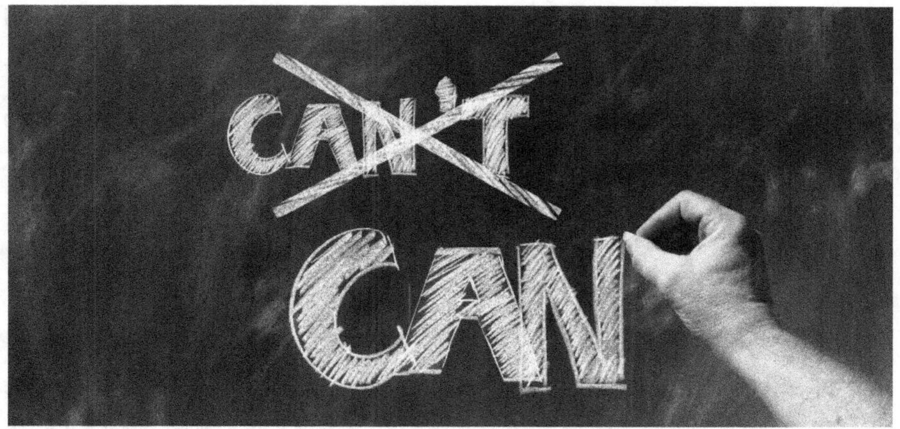

While weight loss is a trending topic in health, achieving it is an uphill task. Considering that a weight program is one of the best things that one does to their bodies, it is important to understand its dynamics. People are getting more aware of the health interventions that will prolong life. Many people choose to lose weight without having solid reasons. However, the reasons do not matter much as the determination to continue in the program.

Cutting some of your weight can make you look better. People who look fit are thought to be cool and they get more friends and social attention. The reward package of weight loss is more than the physical changes. Confidence comes when one is sure about their image. Weigh loss can, therefore, be the gateway to improved relationships between people. This makes you have a thing less to worry about n your life. People who don't have to think over their image tend to concentrate their efforts and attention to careers and other aspects of life.

There are thousands of reasons to lose weight. They don't have to be scary to make one consider getting into a program. All an individual needs are facts about lifestyle choices. Some people are not moved by the fear-inflicting statistics about obesity although a good number of people benefit from the same. The elderly people who desire to live longer may be concerned about osteoarthritis and would be willing to intervene. Younger people would rather lose weight for the aesthetic value.

Weight loss is a tool that can make life easier. Preventing joint damage by shedding some pounds will help you tolerate more exercise. This means that you will enjoy hitting the gym and end up losing more weight. Some such benefits of weight loss are not only instant but they have a cumulative value. As an intervention, weight loss has the potential to reverse disease processes. Progressive blockage of arteries due to cholesterol deposition can be halted by reducing sources of fat in the diet. This prevents a heart attack and the hardening of blood vessels. Breathing problems can be solved by lose weight. Fat deposits in the chest region put pressure on the lungs causing difficulties in breathing. Sleep apnea which is potentially harmful could be caused by obesity.

The immune system invariably needs a boost to function optimally. Fat is a source of inflammation and the load is transferred to the immune system. The individual ends up misusing the immune cells that would otherwise help fight off infections. A weight program can help one get back the ability to neutralize dangerous toxins and germs that enter the body through various portals. This ability to protect the body is an important determinant of healthy living across all age groups.

Obesity is a problem which causes more problems. Finding the motivation to keep going even when the odds are against you is necessary to get the life of one's desire. Giving up shouldn't be an option since there are many alternatives to getting to lose weight. However, the nature of the human body seems to be resistant to change. This is unfortunate for weight programs because the aim to get some significant change. Copying mechanisms work hard to get the body to adapt to the new changes. When the individual gets used to the change in routine, going on remains to be the only easy option.

Any major event in the life of an individual is likely to receive criticism. Weight loss critics deal a blow to the psyche of one struggling to get healthier. The stigmas associated with being obese can really harm one's social life. People who quit weight loss programs give in to these challenges. These are some of the external factors that crush the hope on someone who had set off well in weight loss interventions. Entry into a weight loss program is the hardest part of the decision to change your weight. After the initial adjustments, you will get used to it. People who don't know this aspect will give up quickly. They think that they will continue with the challenges for longer than the time taken to benefit.

Unless there is an inherent medical problem that prevents one from losing weight, the results of a weight loss intervention plan should be seen soon. Some people want to exercise and lose weight instantly. This works for some but not all the people. If one doesn't see any changes after a couple of months, they are likely to surrender. To avoid this, an individual has to look for the program that fits them. Instead of giving up, it is wiser to seek help from a professional who knows more about the diet or exercise.

You can get to a program that requires you to quit your favorite foods and it works for you. The incessant cravings driving you crazy will become your point of weakness. The approach in such a scenario would be to find healthy alternatives that will still keep you on track. Better still; get a diet that allows you to eat things that please your taste buds and you will go a long way. Diets alone for weight loss can be stressing. Unless you supplement with exercises, you will likely be required to choose a very strict unpleasant diet.

Understanding the basic principles of weight loss can help demystify assumptions that hinder progress. Being well informed helps an individual summon more energy to get going. For instance, weight loss will be achieved only if you end up with fewer calories in the body at the end of the day. This can be done by reducing the intake or burning more calories. By grasping the concept, you will appreciate staying hungry sometimes. It will also help in decision making in terms of which foods to eat and the type of exercises to undertake. Subsequent chapters will offer feasible plans to mentally motivate one when they are losing weight.

OVERCOME FEARS

Fear is a setback that can cripple your weight loss efforts. People fear things that are strange to them and tend to avoid doing such things. Apart from the techniques involved, there are fears of consequences that are associated with weight loss programs. Either you fear to lose too much weight or more commonly to regain weight after losing. Altogether, there is the fear of failure in achieving the desired goal. Fear is part of life and it instructs one to be careful in doing things. However, too much fear could be hindering you from advancing in anything.

One thing that one is sure of is that there will be some level of success. Whether the success will be significant to one's health can be questionable. Fearing that you will put back the lost weight after several months or years of exercising can be discouraging. The dread is a reality since it can happen but it shouldn't be in your mind all

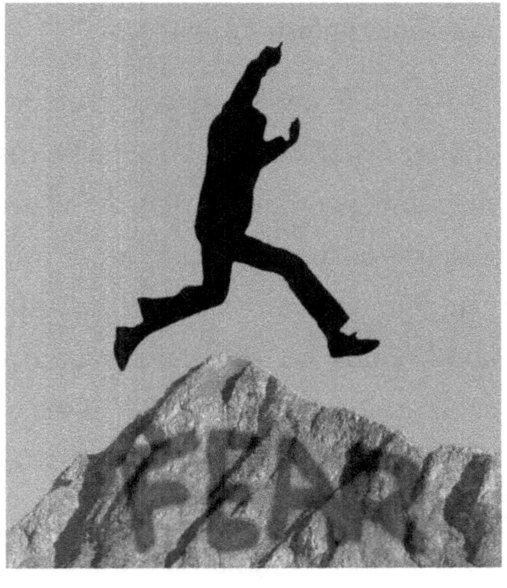

the time. Even expecting the worst is good for preparing for it but it is pointless to be obsessed with negativity. It takes a lot of bravery to face the fears and push them aside. Once you tame the fear, you can over-rule its power over you.

It is not uncommon to find people with a great task to lose much weight fearing that they will always go back to their previous state. They are so used to seeing their bodies in such a shape that they doubt if they can maintain a different weight. People who fear that they won't make permanent changes in their weight have a typical behavior of keeping different sizes of clothes. The expectation is that they will find over-sized clothes handy when they regain weight. Nothing kills one's psyche as the belief that changes are temporary. The mere thought that you will get back to square one is not in keeping with the rigorous exercises that lead to weight loss. Slowly and progressively you will give up on some tasks at the gym. You will prefer to do things that won't strain you since there is the lack of motivation. Poor exercising techniques will contribute to poor weight loss thus confirming your fears.

The attitude needs to be worked on until one appreciates the small changes and becomes rational. Losing weight through exercising helps one get more muscle than fat. The more muscular you get, the easier it becomes to burn more calories. Adopting such an attitude can help one who is perpetually afraid that their efforts aren't any good. Emotions and behavior are different and they should stay separated in the individual. Associating emotions with behavior doesn't work well in weight loss. The love of some unhealthy but delicious foods should be separated from the actual act of cooking such foods. Emotional eating leads to weight gain because of the poor food choices. Fear and anxiety can be interpreted as hunger leading to unnecessary eating.

Every undertaking can have an associated risk and the where the benefits outweigh the risks, you should take a chance with the task. Although there is the possibility of regaining weight, the immediate and long-term benefits of weight loss should be the driving factors. The health gains for weight loss are far much bigger than the probable bad outcomes. Knowing what is at stake can help reduce your fears since you will be able to do some tradeoffs. Trying might work but not trying won't work at all.

Changing the perception may end up being the rational viewpoint. In dealing with your fears you need to look at things differently. For instance, regaining weight is not completely bad and it's certainly not a failure. In the obsession to lose weight, overdoing it may push you towards a lower side of the scale. After all, you don't need to lose so much weight as to get undernourished. In such instances, it is worth celebrating some

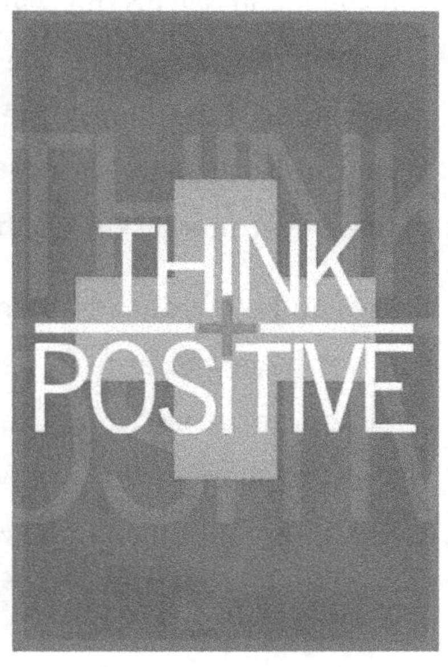

weight gain. Regaining weight inappropriately simply means that it is time to try some other diet and exercise. This should be an interesting time since you don't get to a point of monotony. Some of the mistakes that one does end up unnoticed until one thinks of giving up. Binging even once in a while is as dangerous as eating large amounts of food over time. Therefore, make an audit of your lifestyle and remove anything that can lead to bad outcomes. Once you are sure that everything is clear, your fear will be resolved.

You may think that you lack the motivation to go on but the truth of the matter is that you fear something. Find out the real reason why you are avoiding doing something. Most of the time, it is a form of belief that you hold so dearly that you think you are not motivated. An example of this is one who fails to hit the gym because they fear that they will expose their bodies and get embarrassed. To find out if it is a lack of motivation or the fear of shame, change the environment. You can find a private place where you get to be alone and see if you will do the regular exercises. If fear is the cause of lack of motivation, make ultimate changes to your daily routine. The daily walk can be done during the time when you go to pick up your kid from school. You can choose to take the stairs to your office instead of the elevator and skip an after-lunch snack.

Once you have your fears under check, don't postpone a healthful habit or have excuses. To be successful, you need to keep doing it until you get used to it. The more you perform the exercises, the higher the chances that you will outlive your fears. Live to enjoy the health intervention and you will be motivated to do it every day.

HABIT VS WILLPOWER

We need the willpower to undertake some tasks. However, sustaining it is so difficult that we are likely to fail. Habits, whether good or bad, will end up forming much of our daily activities. This means that willpower without habits is almost pointless. We need both the willpower and habit forming to do new tasks but we need the habits more for long-term projects. Habits die hard and can be the only option when one is idle. This is in sharp contrast to willpower which depends on many factors. No wonder, you may be too tired to do something at the end of the day because the events of the day drained your willpower.

Why Habit is more important than Willpower

Habits are powerful when you are tired and lack the willpower to do anything constructive. You may be stressed up or unhappy and you will find solace in doing the things you have learned and practiced over time. If you have a habit of hitting the gym, for example, you won't feel the burden of putting on the gym gear. In fact, you will do the habit to reduce desperation. It is therefore important to select a healthful habit that will help improve your lifestyle. Good habits are more rewarding and attracting even if they seem to get tougher. The reward system is free from later regrets when you do something positive.

Many habits are loops of repetitive behavior that we adopt along the way. A habit may be something cool you saw someone else doing and you decided to take on it. The loop begins with a cue that signals the need to do the habit. The stimulus is anything like the environment or a sense of free time. When you get the right stimulus and occasion it with a routine, it simply becomes a habit. Sometimes you can't explain why you always act in a certain way when you see or smell something. It is a habit and you do it with the subconscious mind.

Since habits are automatically undertaken, there is a considerable efficiency that is associated with them. For instance, you don't need to get a physical reward when you want to perform a habit. To get the willpower to act on anything, you may need a form of an encouragement. Removing the incentive deals a blow to your willpower and you end up sliding back into an unhealthy lifestyle. Forming a habit will ensure that you not only conserve resources but also get to sustain the healthful action.

Healthy choices are not necessarily the best of choices. A cookie is sweet to the tongue and you would rather take sweet foods when stressed up. If you have the willpower, you may convince yourself that you'll workout immediately after the unhealthy habit. This is a form of compensation which has the potential to help the individual. However, how about forming a habit of taking a smoothie when stressed? It may not be as sweet as high-calorie foods but habits can support such a healthy decision.

Anything can fit into the habit loop and it doesn't have to make sense. Instead of going to the office using the elevator, you may just mindlessly decide to walk the stairs. Willpower will not promote such a decision because there is a simpler but unhealthy option. Such things are best left to the power of a habit. You will find it easy to use the stairs even when tired because you have formed a routine of doing so. Habits overrule the willpower since they get a preference and are deeply rooted in the cognitive function of the brain.

BAD HABITS YOU SHOULD QUIT RIGHT NOW

People begin doing things and end up forming habits that may be unhealthy. Breaking a habit needs firm decision and the knowledge of its impact on health can help. There are benefits to stopping some of these habits earlier since they have an influence on your longevity. Such habits like a fast eating pace that must be stopped immediately may seem harmless. A closer look will reveal how dangerous they are to the health of an individual.

Eating too quickly

Eating quickly to finish the plate in less than 5 minutes does more harm than benefit in your diet. The rush time does not allow for adequate mastication, an important first step of eating. You need to chew food well to expose a larger surface area of the particles for subsequent action of the stomach and intestinal juices. Gulping food at the fast rate will lead to indigestion and a feeling of discomfort. If you had planned to hit the gym later on the day, consider the gym trip cancelled.

You will end up eating a lot of food in the short time because you depend on the brain's satiety centre to give the stop signal. The excess food will add an extra load of calories to the body which cannot exercise efficiently. You should learn to eat slowly and let the food get digested properly. This will help you get the maximum nutrition from a small amount of food.

Skipping your Breakfast

Many people who try to lose weight make a habit of skipping breakfast. This is detrimental to the very efforts of staying healthy. The night fast and the surge of stress hormones like cortisol require you to provide energy from the breakfast. Your metabolic demands are highest in the morning and keep increasing with activity towards lunch time. Skipping the breakfast will make the metabolism sluggish. You will get tired easily on moderate exertion and when it's time for lunch you will eat a lot of food to compensate. The impulse to overeat at lunch will cause you to store calories and gain weight.

Cutting on Sleep

Sleep is very essential for the normal functioning of the body. It is supposed to be a time of complete rest. Cutting sleep to less than 7 hours will affect you negatively and add on the sleep debt which must be paid. You will lack the energy to do healthy activities because you will struggle with keeping awake while at work. A lack of sleep leads to postponement of duties to cover for the insufficiency. The immunity is replenished when we sleep and people who sleep less end up hurting the immune system.

Pessimism

It is expected that an individual will not trust everything that comes their way. However, it shouldn't get to pessimism and negativity because this will not support healthy activities. It is important to stop being negative all the time if you are beginning on a project. Failure should be seen as a chance to improve on your efforts. This will help you go on with tough projects like a weight loss program. Bad thoughts fed on the mind for a long time induce stress and depression. The physical and mental effects of pessimism are too much and are better prevented than dealt with.

Snacking endlessly

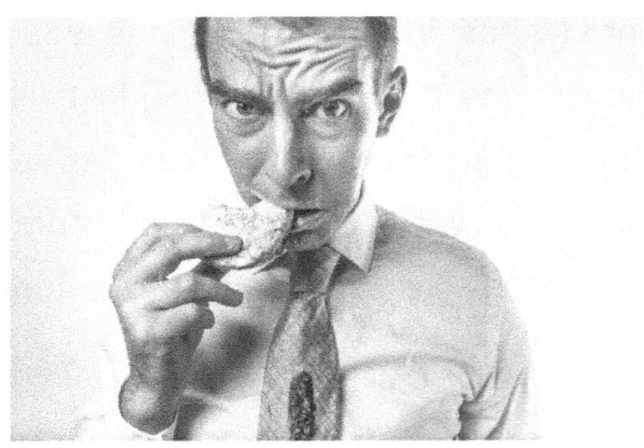

While people can successfully cut on excessive eating, it becomes a poor habit if it is replaced with snacking endlessly. Taking snacks too frequently may end up being more dangerous than over-eating during your regular meals. You should stop snacking when you are not hungry and this will reduce the frequency of eating. Wait for the hunger signal before you eat and when you eat, choose healthy snacks.

Stop watching too much TV

Sitting in your living room scrolling through the TV channels will make you physically inactive. It will do you better to practice relaxation exercises like Yoga to calm yourself after a long day at work. Watching the TV is associated with unhealthy choices. Since you already feel like a loser, you will find your way to eating more fatty high-calorie food. You should limit your TV time and dedicate more time to visiting friends or doing an interesting hobby.

Stressful Habits

Stress hormones are meant to help you prepare for a fight or a flight. They, therefore, lead to an increase in the blood sugar and slow down the gut processes to allow for other priorities like maintaining the brain and heart function. The result is an increased load of calories which need to be burned. Stop stressful habits that jeopardize your health by switching to more friendly options. Learn to cope with stress by first avoiding the cause and then stay cool. This will help prevent diabetes and other health conditions that would otherwise make it difficult for you to maintain healthy habits.

HABITS YOU SHOULD START TODAY

If you are going to quit the bad habits, you need some form of a replacement. The habits to inculcate in your daily life should be healthful and achievable. Since you can't handle all the healthy habits at once, you will need to advance slowly. The aim is to set new norms that will become part of your culture. A successful new habit is bound to encourage you to go for more until you make a complete turnaround.

Goal Setting

The first step or habit that you should begin today is to learn to set goals. Everything you do will make more sense if you have a goal. Goal setting determines the endpoint of an activity and a beginning of another action. The closer you are to the set goals, the more you feel like you will achieve the target. You don't have to set up long-term goals at the beginning. Just be fair to yourself and begin with small steps. After hitting the target, you can advance slowly and set up higher targets. Goals help individuals to set up the path to success.

Walk more and Drive Less

The car is good for convenience. However, you can choose to walk to the local store and only drive when traveling over long distances.

Walking counts as part of workouts. Some people burn all their target calories by walking alone for a few blocks every day. Through walking, you improve your muscle strength and get to tolerate more exercise. This will reduce the risks of heart diseases that arise from an excess of cholesterol buildup in the vessels. The good thing about walking is that you don't need extra resources like the gym equipment. You get healthy without having to break the bank.

Go Green

Green foods are full of vital nutrients and one can get maximum benefit by changing their diet. You should make a habit of choosing greens over other types of food. This is to 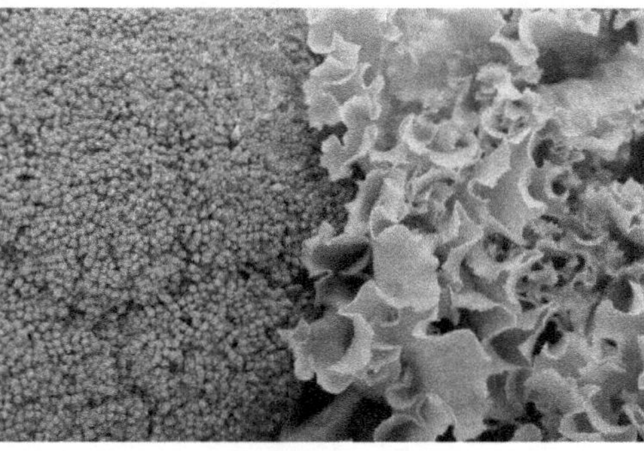 ensure that the greater percentage of your food is made up of vegetables and fruits. Such foods are excellent sources of roughage, enough carbs, minerals, and vitamins. The breakfast can be in the form of a smoothie made of green leaves of healthy veggies like kales, spinach, and broccoli. If you want to take fats for an added source of energy, you will have choices like the avocado and plant oils.

Drink Water when Thirsty

Soda and diet drinks have a lot of sugar which makes them sweet. The sugar rush brings a short-lived good feeling and the health effects are unfavorable. Make a habit of drinking mineral water whenever you are thirsty. This will quench your thirst and ensure that you end u with more minerals in the system. It takes a lot of restraining to learn to choose water over soda but it becomes easier after a few trials. The feeling that you are making a new healthful habit is great and encouraging.

Love Sleep

The daily hustle should not interfere with your sleep pattern. It is time to focus on your health and be more productive. Respecting bedtime and taking a break from the social media and other issues 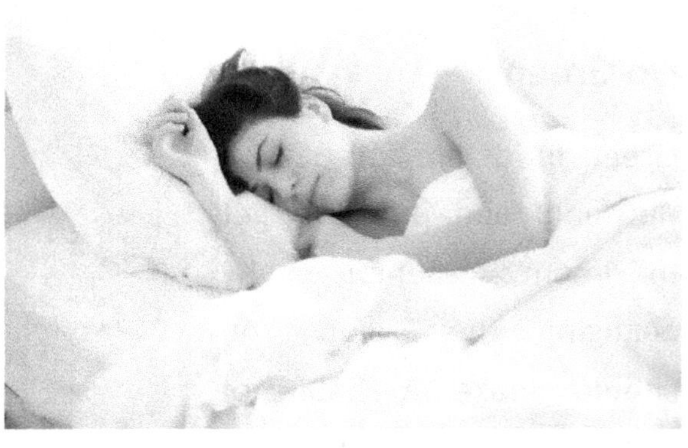 at night will help your sleep life. It is possible to get the adequate amount of sleep if you plan your day well and ensure that everything ends at a time that allows you to sleep for 8 hours. If you choose 10 pm, make it a habit to always sleep at the same time and you will wake up fresh for the day.

TRACK YOUR HABIT

When you've made a healthy choice you need to do everything to keep it. This is the hardest part of living healthfully. Circumstances surrounding you can cause you to forget the habit and you go back to the first step. To avoid this, you should track your habit and follow it until it becomes unshakably strong. Building the habit needs a constant check to note the strengths and the weaknesses of the individual. Without tracking, you can't have a progress report which is useful in making the necessary changes to improve your habits.

Habit tracking is a habit that needs to be learned as well. It is as simple as simply keeping a log of the daily activities but with very strong influences in your habits. Every day, you want to ensure that you didn't miss something regarding the habit. Having the ability to consistently complete the log is as good as doing the habit. You can track multiple habits at the same time and derive a single conclusion. The log should have a provision for both learning and unlearning of habits. This way, you always get motivated that you are in the right direction.

Track the habits that you do on a regular basis. The habits that need to be given a priority are those which mean much to you. Remember that they may be mundane to other people but are very special to you. Using the willpower, form habits and keep the progress on paper until you get convinced that there is no provision for sliding back. As the willpower wanes, the habit gets stronger as evidenced by your developing consistency. This encouragement can only come after you successfully keep the habit journal.

You can only keep a track of a habit that is achievable. There is no point trying to log a habit of running for 3 kilometers when you have been inactive for long. Get to as low as recording a few hundred meters of running. You would rather surpass the target than always find the journal record negative. The effort should be commensurate with your ability and allow for some space for improvement. If you find that you are battling with meeting the target, scale down on the habit task until when you can achieve more comfortably.

Be a regular doer of the habit so that you have something to look forward to tracking. Repetitive behavior becomes ingrained in you a level of automaticity is sparkled. You won't have to keep a reminder that it is time to record your habit progress. The habit tracking act is a form of self-accountability. This way, you can't cheat because you don't have to unlike when you are required to report your progress to someone else. Being responsible for your own actions will reinforce the habits and ensure that you keep doing it over an extended time.

HABIT TRACKING SHEET

Your track sheet is divided into daily goals with entries of the achievement. Focusing on the smaller picture helps you get into finer details. The larger picture will build up without you feeling overwhelmed. An instant progress report on choosing healthy meals, working out, or learning something new helps you feel that you are in control of your health. The need to do more comes after you have hit the daily targets. Small multiple goals will turn into a big final goal of staying healthy. The end-result is embedded in the daily reports.

There are many ways to keep track of your habits. Mobile apps seem to work for some people who know how to use the apps. If they don't work for you after trying a couple of the apps, you can go old school and jot down on a paper. The point is to have somewhere reliable to record your habit details. In the daily planner, the entry can be broad as whether or not you did the habit or more detailed as you will find convenient. Spreadsheets can also do the job well and can be coupled with apps.

For every habit, choose a goal and decide on how you will achieve it in the long run. Think deep into the project and formulate a daily action that will build towards the ultimate goal. This is what you will record in the diary every day. The habits could be multiple or related to the goal and they should be part of the records. Unrelated habits can find their place in another journal book entry to help you stay focused on a goal at a time. This is only for convenience although most of the time, the different habits are learned at the same time.

The habit tracks can help you plan ahead in terms of what you will eat during the day or when you will walk your dog. This helps you to set everything in order and have the healthy options on demand. Being planned makes much difference when your day is full of many possible bad habits. If you plan to eat more greens, you will form a habit of visiting the grocery store after work. This will be recorded in the habit track and later followed by whether or not you actually ate the greens. The same form of habit follow-up applies across different goals.

A reflection on the day's activities will help in evaluating the habits. Were your actions worth the struggle? Could you have done any better? What did you omit in the habit? Such questions can help you during the end-of-day evaluation of the habit track sheet. Make a note of how you feel after achieving the task. After some time, you should be in a position to gauge your progress and how far you are away from the target. Improvements and adjustments should be part of the evaluation with the mission and the vision ever keeping you on your toes.

Print the weekly habit tracking sheet below to track your daily habits;

Weekly Habit Tracking Sheet							
Day	**1**	**2**	**3**	**4**	**5**	**6**	**7**
Wake up early							
Drinking a glass of water as soon as got up							
Morning run							
Eat more vegetables							
Watch less TV							
Walked through the stairs to office							
Meditation							
Eat only when hungry							
Sleep early							
Work towards weight loss goal							
Completed daily workout routine							
Aligned to dietary rules							

SET ACHIEVABLE OBJECTIVES

Many people who want to lose weight get excited and they want to achieve much in a short time. This may seem as an encouragement but actually ends up discouraging the individual when the goals are not achievable. You have to target something that is feasibly attainable. Your body can't take a too drastic weight loss and you have to be aware of it. If possible, think small and surpass your targets rather than get discouraged by underachievement. The measurement on the weighing scale should not be used as an indicator of goal achievement. You could be losing weight but you are still stuck on unhealthy habits which can lead to regaining of weight. The setting of goals outside the weight measurement is more effective in weight loss programs since it focuses on the holistic well-being of the individual. For instance, instead of targeting to lose 50 pounds, you should aim at participating in a challenging event such as a 5000 meters run. There is a high chance that once you finish the run, you will have slashed off a junk of calories.

In weight loss motivation, you don't have to try so hard. You just need to keep going and this means that all you need is enough time to burn some calories. Setting realistic goals will ensure that you don't over-exercise even when your body clearly says no. Weight loss fans need to get their bodies in sync with the program so that the natural processes of the body help you get the most out of minimal time and energy expenditure. It is a clever way to make the body tune to your needs. Sometimes the body needs a break and no matter how hard you struggle, you won't achieve much. During such moments, you have to obey your body and rest for a few days. When you resume, you'll

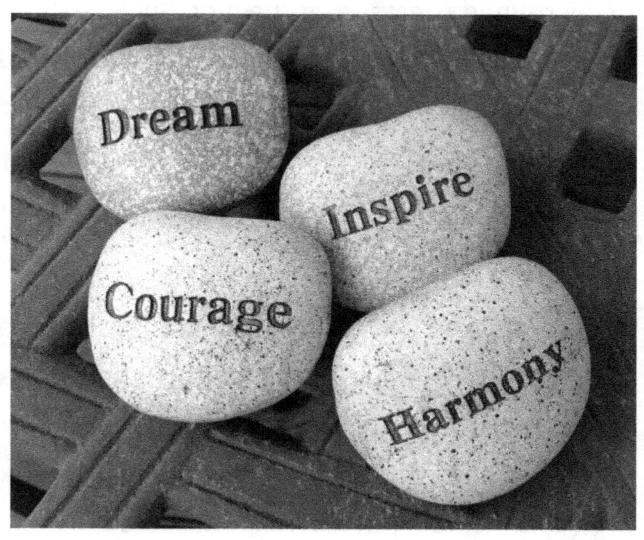

be shocked at how much you can achieve. This way, motivation runs a natural course and you end up benefiting without straining. Trying too hard and failing will kill your psyche and you might find that you are gaining more weight than you intended to lose.

While it is not advisable to set unrealistic goals, you should be serious about the ones you have set. Begin with why you want to lose weight. After you are clear about the motives, write down the specific goals together with their timelines. The laid down goals will help you set up a plan of action which is very important in weight loss. For every pound you desire to shed, there is something different that you must do out of your daily routine. This is part of setting realistic goals because as you write down you'll try to figure out if it is something that you can actually achieve. The aim is to find a suitable workout and diet plan that you are sure you can adhere to. Deciding on what you will do to make your aims real will get you to a point of prescribing a plan such as cardio exercise thrice weekly and strength training on alternate days. In a similar manner, you can choose to cut on all refined sugars from the diet. Such goals will actually make you lose weight without much hustle. Being organized will help you in tackling a goal at a time which is more effective than taking on many weight loss tasks at once. Once you are done with an objective, you can progressively handle more and more until you achieve the appropriate weight loss.

Stay committed with the goals and if possible you should find a way of reminding yourself of the cause. Whenever a temptation to lose hope creeps around, the reminder will keep you going. There are many reasons why you would want to continue in the weight loss program including preventing diseases such as diabetes and heart diseases. You also need to keep fit and presentable. Associating a weight loss intervention with a pleasant feeling is a powerful motivation tool. Every time you feel you have reached the end of the rope, the good feeling you had at the gym should rejuvenate your efforts. Reinforcements are necessary when you are doing a form of exercise that takes much energy. Remember that at first, your body will have a lot of changes with minimal exercising but you will come to a plateau phase. At the plateau, you have to do something extra to get similar results in the weight loss program.

There are extrinsic and intrinsic sources of motivation and both are equally effective. Intrinsic motivation comes from you while extrinsic motivation comes from others. You can exercise because your doctor advised you to do so and that forms the extrinsic sources of motivation. However, if you exercise because you want to accomplish something such as a feeling, it becomes intrinsic motivation. Intrinsic motivation helps one to choose healthful habits which make the individual feel good about their health choices. Similarly, one will choose a habit to stay healthy if they are concerned about what people will see or say about them.

Immediately after one has set goals to achieve weight loss, the extrinsic motivation will give the head start. You will choose to leave that lunchtime snack because of the external pressure to lose weight. Sue these sources of motivation to prepare and even research on the best way forward. Decide on the small things to do or not do so as to get to your goals. Plunging into the weight loss program by relying solely on the external motivation will not only lead to the poor setting of goals but also disappointment from underachieving. The extrinsic motivation can lead to the development of the intrinsic motivation because it helps you understand the health choices better.

Use the intrinsic motivation to commit to a full-scale weight loss program. Having a firmer intrinsic form of motivation will help you succeed in weight loss. If you feel great after making a choice not to eat food with refined sugars or high-fat content, you are more likely to continue with the habit. Developing the intrinsic motivation is easy when you are enlightened. Simply identify what makes you feel good and set realistic goals. Short term goals are easy to achieve and offer a lasting satisfaction. You can go as low as setting a one-hour goal, achieve it and set more. Keeping a journal can help foster your internal motivation. Confidence in your abilities to achieve the unthinkable will improve with time.

PRIORITIZE HEALTHFUL LIVING

New resolutions on healthy living are welcomed with a lot of passion and zeal. However, one finds it hard to keep working out or follow a diet plan. The reason is most likely a lack of prioritization. The secret to getting motivated in weight loss interventions is to make your life a priority over work and other aspects of life. From the outset, doing this is a challenge because of today's setting. You have to rush to work and occasionally squeeze in a snack to boost your energy at lunchtime. Such factors do not give you an easy time to live a healthful life. If you must make daily healthy choices, you must be committed and consistent.

Begin with the basics by making a decision that you want a better life. Look at the bigger picture where the choices you make today will make a positive impact in your future life. Avoid fast foods where possible and go through the process of preparing your food. When you go to the grocery store, buy more healthy foods and have a meal plan as early as a week before. People who know what they plan to eat earlier will make arrangements to look for that particular food item. You will be surprised at how much nutrition you can gain from the diet if you have a plan. Fast foods are usually loaded with calories and are limited in the ability to provide nutrition.

If you plan to lose weight by working out, schedule it in your daily activities. Gym time should not depend on your moods so that you only workout when you like. It should be like going to work;

something that is part of your schedule and cannot be replaced by other activities. At the gym, find something that gives you the desire to exercise. You can have a friend or a mate who 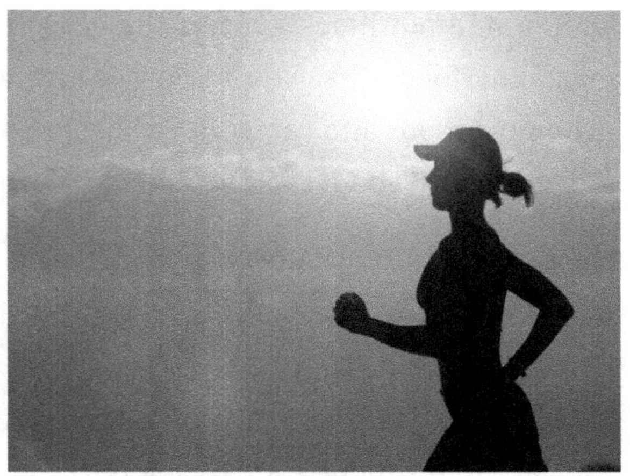 accompanies you to workout but you should be independent and understand that the exercises are meant to make your life better. This way, you always show up regardless of the circumstances.

Trivial things matter in healthful choices. If you walk up the stairs, you'll probably be inconvenienced but end up healthy. You can choose to park your car at the furthest end of the store so that you have to do some extra walking. You can also make it a point to take back the shopping cart into the store instead of letting the attendant do so and you will be another step nearer to weight loss. Utilize every opportunity that presents itself before you to make a healthful choice. It may be cumbersome but you are sure to get used to it if you know the value of what you are doing.

The environment can have a negative impact on your choices. Friends and close associates can influence your decisions and if they do so negatively, you have to choose between them and your health. Don't worry about being lonely because you'll need to lead a longer quality of life if you want to enjoy their company. When you get to your kitchen what do you first see? Change the kitchen environment so that you have no option but to choose healthy food. Stock the kitchen with all the nutritious goodies that you want. Find alternatives to unhealthy foods that you crave because you were used to them. Group the foods into categories of healthy foods and those that you are not certain about their benefits.

Sleep hygiene contributes to a great percentage of healthful living. If you have to doze off at work, you will have to postpone gym time to finish unattended work. You'll also be forced to buy a quick fix food 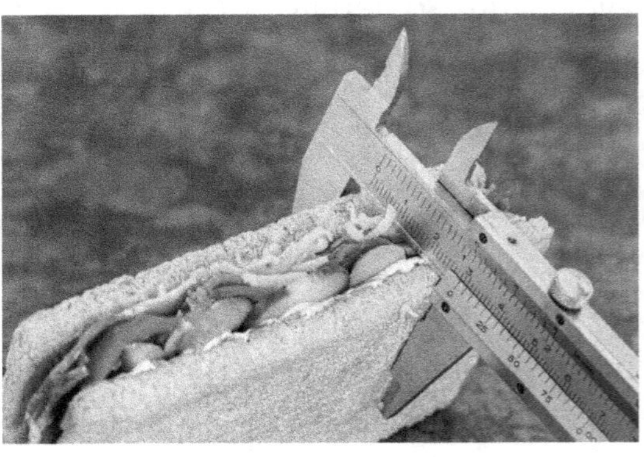 since you want to catch up with lost time. To be effective in the healthy habits, you need to have a good night's sleep. Quality sleep optimizes the body systems so that you don't have problems with digestion and absorption which can lead to issues with the energy required to exercise. Sleep at specific times and aim at getting at least 6 hours of sleep every day. The more sleep, the better but too much will definitely ruin your day. The muscles need to relax before you subject them to another form of exercise. Resting the body is not enough to renew all the systems and sleep is the only time to achieve this optimization. Prioritize sleep and reduce excitement just before bed so that you don't have trouble sleeping.

Reduce the sources of stress in your life to as minimum as possible. There are things that you can do without in your life and those should be the first to strike off. You may need to perform relaxation exercises such as yoga to release some of the excess stressors. Relaxation exercises have the benefit of also helping with weight loss. You don't have to overwork to impress your boss. Just work smart and let your life come first before other things.

Leisure should count as part of the time to get some health benefit through the activities you love doing. It should not be the time to sit by the TV and eat; try to recover some gym time you may have lost during the week. Alternatively, you can schedule the weekend and free time to use in working out routinely. This will help you stay sober while maintaining the hard-earned health benefits. Portable training equipment can give you more freedom and utility. You can easily pull out your training gear during leisure and make the free time count. If you have the option, always prioritize to choose a course of action that will help you in achieving the best health.

APPRECIATE ACCOMPLISHED TASKS

Weight loss takes a focus on changing the behavior that leads to good outcomes. However, the outcome may not be according to your expectations. The best you can do to ensure that you stay optimistic is to appreciate every little accomplishment. Don't let the reward determine your happiness but enjoy the good moments when they come. Small changes should make you feel as good as big changes and they should be recognized as a success. Many people get discouraged when all they can put forth after days of exercise is a few pounds lost. The desire to achieve more is influenced by how you appreciate little efforts in your life.

Compassion can be cultivated by self-appreciation. Think about how far you have come and how efficient you have converted your body into a calorie burning machine. There are things that you either couldn't do before or had a hard time doing. You may not have shed many calories but the fact that you can tolerate more exercise should be a call for celebration. Be grateful that you can move easier, faster, and better than before even if your shape is not yet the best. You may have been unable to stay without a soft drink but now you always quench your thirst with water. That is a big gain and it should not be compared to the scale benefits.

Loving yourself the way you are will be a great step in getting your own approval. People may not appreciate you but if you already love yourself you won't have a problem. Weight loss

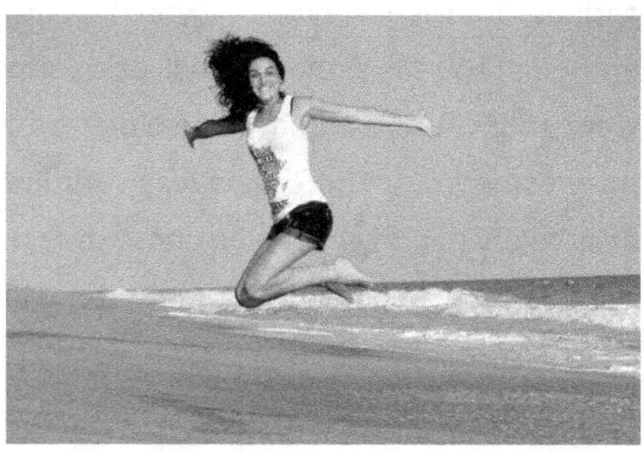

is just one factor in getting the life of your desire. Sometimes it comes early and sometimes it takes quite a lot of effort and time to achieve it. Believe that you have the ability to achieve what you want and be thankful that you are yourself. Figures on the scale will come and go but you will always remain to be you. Be satisfied with your inner self and then work on your goals. Hating your shape, weight, or figure will not motivate you to work any harder than actually discourage you. Remember that for sustainable changes, the motivation needs to come from within and not extrinsically.

A person who mistakenly thinks that they must lose weight to get an approval will end up being distressed. The worst that can happen is that you associate exercising or dieting with negativity. If this happens, be sure to have problems with doing anything that is geared towards securing a better health. Simply appreciate the being that you are and use the exercises and eating right to get to a better place. Healthy choices should not be a punishment for who you are. They should be a form of reward to you and therefore worthy to be undertaken.

Always look for something positive to keep you focused on the big deal. The body can play tricks on you and even gain weight after serious intensive workouts. If you depend on the scale for victory you immediately realize that you will be doomed. While many people may want to give up, you have to soldier on and remember the far you have come from. There is no way your life will ever remain the same after every healthy habit you chose over the many enticing unhealthy options. Use the down moments to improve on the technique of exercise or dieting. You may need to tweak some little details such as frequencies. Once you are satisfied that you have done everything in your power to keep the right health seeking habits, continue pursuing them.

Motivation can get a boost from a feeling of pride out of accomplishments. There is always someone who will appreciate you. The social media can get you a few likes which will put a smile on your efforts. Weight loss sites will offer an encouragement for your successes. Avoid places that can get you criticized and protect every small effort. Learn to also reward yourself by doing something fun. Food or expensive gifts may not be the best way to reward oneself since they have many limitations. Make it simple but worth remembering so that you have fun without having to break the bank. You could buy a new pair of training suit or learn to cook something new.

Rewards have the ability to cognitively condition positive behavior. This way, you choose to do some form of activity because your brain is wired to anticipate it. The reward needs to be meaningful and maintain the standards of healthful habits. Doing this pushes you to the next level in your goal achievement. You can choose to buy clothes that will confer a new image on you. Part of the reward is to forgive and forget your wrongs. Once in a while, you may find yourself in a fix and you didn't know what to do but to make a compromising choice. It is useful to acknowledge the wrong but you shouldn't emphasize it. Judgmental thoughts can drain your positive gains and kill your morale. Sometimes it does not lead to any significant change if all other factors are constant. The weight loss may stagnate for a few weeks but will resume course if only you continue pressing on.

Improve on the factors that led to poor decisions and try not to repeat them. More importantly, focus on the positives at all times. Don't let the past to form loops in your dieting or exercise plan. When you fail, begin there and work towards attaining the goal once again. Don't have excuses that postpone the program until another time. Seek to achieve progress and not necessarily perfection. Allow for a level of failure but appreciate the successes well.

MAJOR ON STRENGTHS

Our bodies are uniquely different and many people who try to copy others end up failing miserably. A poor choice of the weight loss plan can kill your motivation. The program may be effective in helping one to lose weight but it just doesn't work for you. This means that there are some programs that will fit your needs and you will get a desirable weight loss. Even inside the weight cut programs, there are some aspects that favor an individual and these should be utilized to get the maximum benefit. There are many ways to tackle the weight problem including dieting and exercising. You need to do intense research and get to try out some of the options until you find the best for you.

To be successful you need to find something that encourages you and gives you a reason to continue doing it. It should also be safe and allow for individual adjustment so that you can feel in control. Check that the proposed plan fits your lifestyle. It is important to engage in something that won't be interrupted by financial constraints. Look into the future since possible changes in life events can derange our good weight loss progress. Your current health should also be factored in while choosing the plan because some people can't tolerate high-intensity exercises. They are not excluded from the benefits of exercising since there is always something that can be done. The brisk walks and jogging are not inferior to running if you do it right. The point is to major on your strengths and to use them to your advantage. You don't have to struggle to fit into someone else's shoe- just be you and be content.

Understand all the details of your plan so that you can know where to hinge your efforts. The result of the weight loss program needs to be measurable and

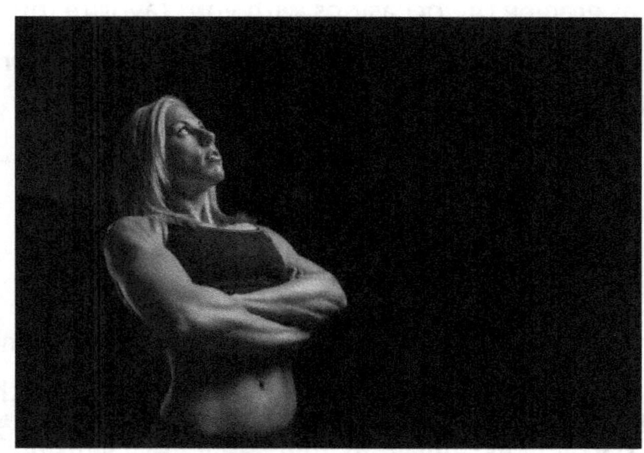

somehow predictable. This is the only way to make a balance of trade and decide on a course of action. Since most plans involve either eating or physical activity, get to know what is on the menu. If you have some vegetarian affiliation, you'll realize that you can use it to get the weight cut. So you will ensure that in the program, you edge towards going vegan.

Sometimes you will be forced to do only some of the tabled weight loss suggestions. The guiding factor in choosing what to do and what to leave should be your perceived strengths. You know yourself better than the weight trainer. No one should impose anything on you because you are the doer and thus the one who gets affected. The many available weight loss options ensure that a busy adult, college student, the elderly, teens, and other categories of people are put into consideration. In all you do, be yourself and appreciate what you can achieve.

Physical activity for weight loss helps in converting one into a calorie burner and improves the mental health. When you are stuck in deciding which way to go, think of an exercise that you will enjoy and stick to then major on it. Look for ways to lengthen the exercise such as gracing the occasions with your favorite music or working out with friends. The biggest challenge comes when starting but when you get used to it you'll have a free ride. Maintain the objective as your steering towards a desirable weight loss. Your fitness level picks up after a few shots at the exercise so you don't have to begin with intense training.

Aerobics, strength, high-intensity interval training, calisthenics, boot camps, balance, and flexibility are some of the classes of exercise types. In aerobics, the individual does continuous moving over some period of time. Swimming, dancing, and running are some examples of aerobic exercises. Most fitness plans will include a form of an aerobic workout as part of their program. Resistance training, weight lifts, sprints, and plyometrics are a good start to increase the muscle strength and power. Sit-ups, push-ups, and pull-ups do not need gym equipment and they are classified as calisthenics. Boot camps simply combine the aerobics and resistance training and are done over a specified time. They are high-intensity exercises swinging from one activity to the other. Balance or stability exercises help in strengthening the muscles and fostering better coordination of the various body parts. An example of a stability exercise is the famous tai chi. Yoga is a relaxation and a flexibility exercise prescription that can be used by people who need to recover or prevent injury.

The options are unlimited as long as you are bent to shed weight. If you are not sure of the exercise of diet that will fit you, feel free to try some first. You'll get to find the program that you can twist and tailor towards your specific demands. Daily training is just as effective as weekly training. While the recommendation is that you not less than 150 minutes of exercising moderately every week, you can surpass the target. This can be done either by increasing the intensity of the workout while maintaining the time or by working out longer. The idea is to burn a certain number of calories every week and lose weight.

During majoring on one's strength, the individual should let the body recover from stress once in a while. The desire to lose more weight quickly can lead to overdoing of an exercise and this is harmful. The same muscles that exercise today will be required to work out tomorrow. Lactic acid and waste metabolites build up in the muscles as you work out. Strains, stress fractures and other injuries occur in people who tend to overwork their bodies. In the long run, resting will prove invaluable because you will be able to exercise all year round. Hormonal imbalances, immune disturbances and depression can occur if you don't get enough rest intervals.

SUPPORT GROUPS

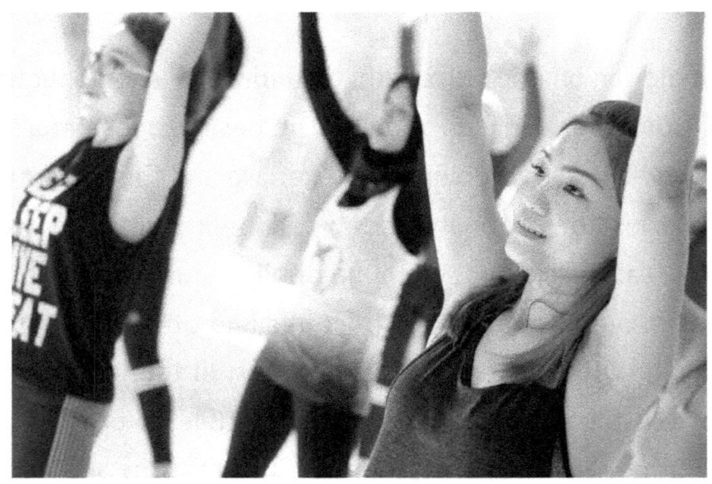

Weight loss is a tolerable journey if the individual gets support on a regular basis. Social support, positive feedback and external sources of motivation are handy when one feels like giving up. People who can offer support include friends, family, and local workout clubs. The closest persons who interact with you should be aware of the weight loss program so that they refrain from tempting you with unhealthy habits. Online support groups are effective in encouraging an individual just as in-person groups do. A strong support community will see to it that you get a boost to your motivation especially in bad times when despair seems to be the only way out.

The advantage of a support group with members who have the same goal is the ability to get your concerns addressed. Some friends or family members may prove difficult and they won't let you do the program because they don't understand your life's objectives. You end up losing the motivation to lose weight when you have constant nagging from people who don't see the value of what you are doing. You may need to join a public gym where your chances of getting a motivation are higher than being alone at home. It is important to have someone to talk to when you encounter problems with your plan. You can get solutions to your issues and be comforted by the fact that many other people have similar issues. Like-minded people give you a reason to be disciplined. Experience and active guidance from other people help you cross the hurdles of weight loss. Coaches and professional weight interventionists can act as your confidants that will help you in every step of the program.

Validation and approval can come from the support community. They help you deal with questions pertaining to the weight loss program. If two or three people talk about doing something you will be convinced that it is the right thing. Doubts of whether you will be fine or succeed in the plan may exist. The people you meet in the social group will help you feel secure and take the risk. Insight, the right perspective, and real experiences are the aspects that improve on your internal motivation. If you fail in some part of the plan be sure to have an attentive ear from the group. They will empathize and make you forgive yourself.

An educated person is an empowered individual. Expert advice from books, websites, and social weight loss communities are instrumental in changing your mindset. Knowing why exactly you should cut on calories from refined sugars is more effective in silencing the cravings for sweet food than simple avoidance. Sometimes one thinks that they are not the right candidates for weight loss because they have tried almost everything. Little details such as the right technique which make all the difference can be learned from others. The thought that you have not exhausted all your weight loss options is inspiring. A great social support is a learning ground that is rich in resources such as principles of success in a particular exercise or diet.

Struggling alone to figure out how to get enough protein in the paleo diet can be a daunting task. However, when people discuss it in a forum such as the social media you get a lot of suggestions. Beginners, as well as veterans, always have something to learn from each another. Groups that invite guests end up ensuring that their members go home holistically trained to handle life matters. A wide base foundation of knowledge is useful in maintaining long-term goals. Participating in the events organized by the social support groups can help reinforce the learned principles.

The strength of a weight loss group is manifested in its ability to keep one accountable. You don't want to disappoint your friends who have walked you through very tricky situations. Constant check-ins motivate your consistency in workouts and strict diet plans because you always anticipate a visit. Weekly weight measurement or use of non-scale victories can help you stay focused on the ultimate prize. The coach or workout friend can make you accountable and they will expect to see you hit the gym every day. You don't have to keep a reminder when you have an accountability partner who makes you look forward to doing healthful habits.

The power in numbers is a survival technique that is deeply rooted in our genes. We feel safer when we participate in an activity that has many people. Harder things can be tried because the participants have the desire to compete favorably. Anxious moments fade off when you have some people accompanying you in the weight loss program. There is a guarantee that someone in the group knows what keeps you motivated. Some people are motivated well enough to continue in the plan until the end when they get the right help. Without this support, an individual is likely to fall off the track at some point. Lone rangers get easily discouraged by life events like the loss of a loved one. One can regain lost weight because of the stresses of life while still going on with the weight loss program. A support group will help you cruise the moments of desperation and get back on track quickly.

Celebration moments are bigger and better when you have people who contributed to your success as part of the crew. In the support groups, you will be celebrating major life accomplishments of many people. Getting the rare recognition of efforts from your peers helps you be rededicated to the cause. You will feel the worth of your actions that may have sacrificed on the time spent with your family and friends. Mixed emotional reactions from people who were used to you could hinder you from the target. Successes should be celebrated well to ensure that you get motivated. Be free with the social group and let them help you when you feel stuck or unsure of something.

EXPECT SETBACKS

Things may go wrong during the weight loss program. People who do not anticipate setbacks are hit hardest when they occur because they don't have a plan to salvage the situation. Problems can come from within the program or as a result of personal issues. A compulsion to binge-eat can be due to feelings of anger or sadness. When you give in to the eating fantasies you end up more depressed since you know that you have an additional calorie burden. Such moments can really work you up until you chose to quit. Unfortunately, the challenges are numerous and frequent in any weight loss program.

The key to ensuring that you are set to counter every setback is to evaluate your vulnerability. Once you identify the triggers you can set effective remedies to help you stay focused on the weight loss goal. The commitment to a diet or an exercise is also a challenge to the individual. Uncertainty can spark fear of change and it will be reflected in your body physically and mentally. People are secure in doing things that they are sure about the outcomes and expectations. Being open for anything should be the way to prepare to get into the program. A good thing like weight loss can be perceived negatively by some people who are in the business of killing your psyche. Such individuals may have an experience in the field and they will try to convince you why you should quit. An individual should have a stand backed up with facts and a hope for a better life. These are the arsenals to prepare you to meet head-on with negativity and pessimism.

Holidays and parties can be really challenging when it comes to maintaining healthy standards. You always get stronger temptations when you want to celebrate with family and friends. Remember that the events are there for a moment and after that, you are left struggling alone. The boss may be out to find faults in your work for some reason and if you are not careful, it will mean bad to your weight loss progress. Before the problem arises, you should have made efforts to mentally solve the possible issues that may hinder your plan. The thought that you have already figured out the problem before it occurs gives you an advantage. Your confidence levels are boosted making you an efficient problem solver.

Anxious people are unlikely to lose and maintain the lost weight for long. They turn to poor comfort strategies such as sweet foods. On the other hand, an individual who is appropriately prepared will look for a solution that makes them even healthier. Since eating is likely to lead to weight gain during stressful moments, you can do square breathing exercises or take a walk. This will only happen if you have decided that you want to stay in the program no matter the situation. Some people who give up on weight loss do so during stressful moments. They take advantage of the setbacks and find excuses for not being in the program.

You can always go back to the basic steps if you feel overwhelmed by the exercise or diet. The initial surge of motivation can wear off slowly and you begin to prioritize other things in life. When you feel that you can't do put any more efforts into the weight loss program, you have probably lost it. Quickly look back and do what you used to do before.

Maybe it was the journal that kept you motivated and happy to work out or do something healthy. Little things like counting the glasses of water you drink every day can rekindle your love for weight loss.

Let your setbacks be moments of reflection and opportunities for self-appreciation. This is the time when you want to remember the reason for joining the weight loss program in the first place. The reasons for the healthful living probably remain constant. The perception may be distorted but remembering the benefits will make you feel that you were on the right track. The next course of action is to get back to the plan usually with more zeal than ever before. If this happens, the setbacks have helped you rather than harmed you. Just accept the ups and downs as part of normal living and continue with the program.

When you get a setback, make sure to survey the damage since it will help in resuscitation. Don't fear to look at the scale when finding out how bad the problem has affected you. It is better to clear the air once for all and get a solution that to be stuck in contemplation. Having facts will help you measure your progress once you are back on track. It can be discouraging to think that you have not lost any weight because you feared to measure your weight. In fact, you get difficulties in starting again unless you are sure of your current standing. Avoid waiting to measure the weight after a couple of exercises. It will delay the process of recovery and lead to more deterioration.

Once you have made an assessment on the pitfall, stop digging for further details which won't help you get back on track. Over-thinking about the matter can always lead to unearthing more discouragements. Silence the inner critic with new goals and begin to work to achieve them. Renewing your mind will involve replacing bad thoughts with good ones. You may need to work harder than before to get back the weight drop. Accept this fact and work until you get the satisfaction that comes with success. A little guilt is allowed as long as it doesn't get you to stress and bingeing. Stop worrying over the past mistakes and have self-compassion. Meanwhile, you should prepare for similar future challenges. Repeat good deeds and you will feel great once again. Exercise patience so that you don't get the drive to set unrealistic goals. Lost time may not be recoverable but regained weight can be lost.

BE OPTIMISTIC

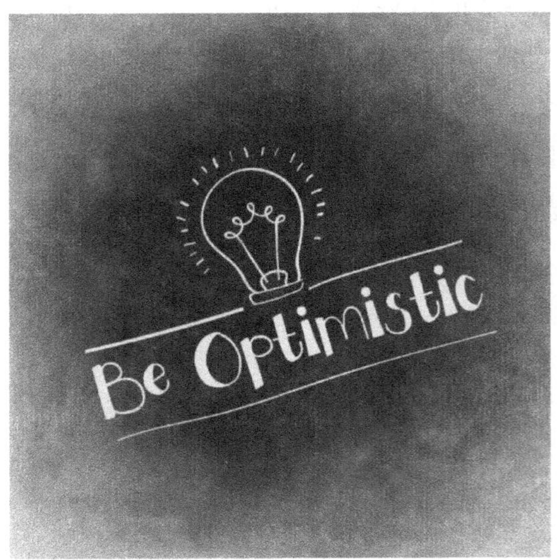

Optimism is a positive thinking tool that builds confidence and helps in goal attaining. When you see things in their best image, you get inspired and lead a happy life. You may have developed a pessimistic attitude towards weight loss especially if you have tried man options that seemed not to work for you. One thing you should be sure of is that you have not tried everything. Let go of the past and get a brand new positive view of the weight loss program. Negativity won't do you any benefit other than complete the destructive process of pessimism.

Getting the bad thought processes out of your mind is a battle that involves introducing new positive thinking in everything you do. It takes a belief that you can get to the desired weight no matter the circumstances. Some weight loss plans such as the HCG will jumpstart your weight loss efforts. You may need to find a starter plan that will put you to a better level if you have been downcast and disappointed before. However, the ultimate tool that one needs to consistently lose weight is optimism. It is found in many people and those who lack it can practice the art of appreciating things without looking for faults. This is important in life and more so in weight loss which is occasioned by a lot of challenges. You want to lose weight but keep falling back to unhealthy habits because of your sedentary job. Sometimes you just have to get a quick fix to get the energy to continue with the day's activities. Junk foods become part of your diet and you are almost powerless about it.

Defeat attitudes from stigma against obese people can make healthy habits almost impossible. When thoughts of desperation orchestrate your weight loss program you may not see the benefits of cutting weight. Everywhere you turn to is a scorn regardless of whether or not you keep doing what is in the weight loss plan. The only way out is to be optimistic that the challenges won't last a lifetime. Use the little positivity that almost everyone is born with to cultivate bigger optimistic perceptions of the environment and the people you interact with.

People can use anything to get a negative self-talk that leads to pessimism. For instance, you could choose to say that you can't lose weight because your parents are overweight and the genes are responsible. Another optimistic individual will decide that they will keep on working hard to lose weight through healthful habits without considering the genes. You may not have made much progress in the scale measurements but you should keep hoping that the small changes will soon make a big difference in the near future. Exercise and dieting are not forms of punishment for being overweight. They are simply healthy and everybody who cares for their longevity should practice them.

Food is a source of fuel for the body and should never be a measure of fun. Friends and activities are sources of fun moments without risking your getting more weight. Willpower is not a determinant of how best you can perform an exercise. Tolerating tough exercises or strict diets takes the skill power of making deliberate moves in and around your life. You identify good habits and plan in advance to have them as part of your weight loss plan. Being positively minded will lower the chances of dropping from the weight programs by improving on your self-image and approval. The mental journal entry should be more of the good things that you managed to achieve that day and not the aspects that you missed, unfortunately.

Believe in your abilities to change every situation that pertains to your weight. First, believe that weight loss is for the best of your life. When you affirm your decision to move the scale pointer you will realize that you deserve to do anything that will make you healthy. The actions to make you happy and healthy become the very actions that lead to weight loss. The belief that you can achieve your goals should be renewed daily. The achievements that you have had before in life can entice your belief in your ability to make better health choices. In fact, weight loss should be viewed as another upcoming victory with the trophy of a disease risk-free life.

Pessimists are afraid of changes because they associate them with a possibility of something going wrong. If you get into a weight loss plan with this notion, you will have trouble coping with bad days. Yet, it is how one reacts to a challenge that matters more than the problem itself. Succumbing to the food cravings is not part of optimism. You should focus on how good you will feel at the next moment just after the craving has passed. Instant rewards are not as great as those that a person works to achieve. Failure comes only when you fail to continue with the program. Otherwise, no matter how many times you skipped to do something healthy you are still on the winning side if you don't give up.

There is no provision for personal blame when you want to keep everything positive. You can choose to view the moments when you lack the drive to run or eat right as holidays. You should have regular intervals of breaks for that matter and for purposes of breaking monotony. The breaks from normal routine will foster your emotional as well as physical strength for the journey to weight loss. Always believe that you are already at the top of the ladder and you will surely reach there. Being optimistic in such a manner that weight loss stops being a challenge will help an individual lose weight. It may take time to develop a positive mind but it is worth the struggle.

DEVELOP ROUTINE AND FIND A ROLE MODEL

Weight loss cannot be achieved through a temporary plan. You have to make a routine change in your life that will accommodate lasting healthful habits. Weight loss motivation can come from the simple act of being organized and following a daily routine. You don't have to repeat doing the same thing in the name of a routine. All you are required to do is have specific times when you want to accomplish certain tasks. With dieting, a routine is so important that it will prevent impulsivity and poor meal choices. Once you have the routine set, you have to commit to it and ensure that you don't miss to do anything or else you will derange the whole plan.

The routine should be easy to formulate and follow so that it becomes interesting. Exciting opportunities are out there to make you healthier. Expect challenges in beginning the plan and be open-minded to any changes that may be needed to make the plan workable. Your whole life will change including the sleep and wake pattern. A good attitude is required to shape the schedule of the life changes. Balancing your job or career, exercising, family, and diet will be important to ensure that you don't overdo one thing at the expense of the other. The weight loss goal will instruct how your routine will run. If you want to target losing a certain weight over a few weeks, the program will likely to be packed. It may strain your efforts but there are benefits that are accrued from a fast weight loss plan. You could decide on a moderate intensity program and while the weight cut may span over some months, you are likely to stick to it.

From the variety of weight loss fitness and dieting options, make a choice that will fit your current lifestyle. Inside the program, have a variety of things that you can do 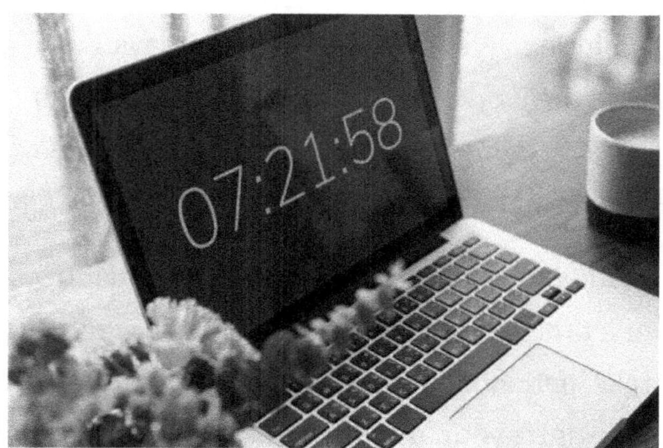 during the time slot reserved for that particular program. You can mix up workouts or skip alternate days to keep you from getting bored by the routine. If you did intense resistance training in a certain day, you can do less the next day for half the time and the shift to aerobics during the remaining period.

Do you have a dedicated room for the exercises? Picking a specific place to perform the workout activities will confer a better adherence to routine. You don't have to do it at the gym although it is better resourced. Set aside some corner at the living room or the office to use for workouts when time catches up with you before you reach the place of choice. Improvise and be creative to get what you want without infringing on other people's space. A walking path at the neighborhood can be utilized for your daily rounds. The point is to make it a place that is easy to access routinely.

Have time limits for the weight loss program in which you assess your progress and set new goals. It should be like moments of refueling your body so you should set the time frames to coincide with when you feel exhausted. Set both long-term and short-term limits with regular intervals. The importance of setting the interval limits is to avoid inconveniences. There are days when you feel like going on with the workouts but you should remember that there are probably other activities waiting for you. The success of the weight loss plan is enhanced by having a routine that is flexible but consistent.

Lasting routines are only possible if you introduce one healthful habit at a time. Your daily routine is in the mental map of your brain. It will take patience and single habit substitutions to reroute the mental map into your desired course. Focusing on more than one habit makes the whole routine complex and almost impossible. You should minimize the moments of failure since they act negatively on your motivation. People give up when they feel overwhelmed by the technicalities of the weight loss programs. To keep your ego rich and attain the goals at the same time, you have to be smart in structuring the routine.

In the plan, identify harmful habits that drain your willpower and find a similar but healthy replacement. Eating a high carb diet before going to exercise may be a good source of energy. However, there are better healthy sources of energy such as fruits. Once you have the right substitute, maintain the gains by removing all the bad options around you. The part of your new routine with difficult tasks can be augmented by having a reward at the end. The reward should be strong enough to motivate you and sometimes you will be forced to bend the strict routine to accommodate it.

A role model can spur your weight loss if you find the right one. Some people have lived through the toughest plateau moments by looking at a picture of their role models for motivation. However, it is good if you can get a role model who is accessible so that you can share with them when you have challenges or when you want to make huge changes in your routine. A friend, colleague or someone who has some experience in the field of weight loss can be a source of inspiration. With the blooming social community on the internet, you can find a very good mentor that will remotely give guidance and encouragement.

The fitness idol helps in reminding one of the need to stick to the best life choice ever- weight loss. Getting motivated can be as easy as desiring to be like someone who is an achiever. Active people offer sound advice since they are well informed of new developments. You can copy some of their activities and integrate them into your routine. People who take shortcuts to reach their goals should not be sued as role models. You should find someone who got to lose their weight through methods that you can practice.

PART 2

THE DIET GUIDE

HEALTHY BODY WEIGHT

It is becoming increasingly important to get a healthy body weight. At the same time, today's sedentary lifestyle makes it hard to achieve this noble task. It is on that note that we offer a solution using our diet program. The easiest way to cut excess calories is to reduce the dietary intake. In this plan, you will learn many hacks to ensure that you not only lose weight but also maintain it. Many people have actually attained a healthy weight only to return to their former state after a few months. This plan adequately covers all the aspects necessary to keep you in shape. Following it will encourage you to lead a healthful life. The health choices stipulated in this book ensure that you have a balance in your diet as you lose weight. You may have tried other weight loss programs before but this one is unique and scientific based.

Many diseases and cancers have been associated with an increased body weight. It is therefore important to look into your weight and make the necessary adjustments to get the benefits of a healthy weight. Although there are additional factors that may be required to trigger a disease process, weight has more influence on your health than most of them. Weight is not just a figure; it is a measure of your health and potential to live longer and happier. Some of the benefits of a healthy weight include lowering the risk of getting diabetes, heart diseases, cancers, and other chronic diseases.

Extra body weight coming from the too much fat deposition in the fat stores leads to lipid metabolism problems. These problems include stroke, heart diseases, gallstones, 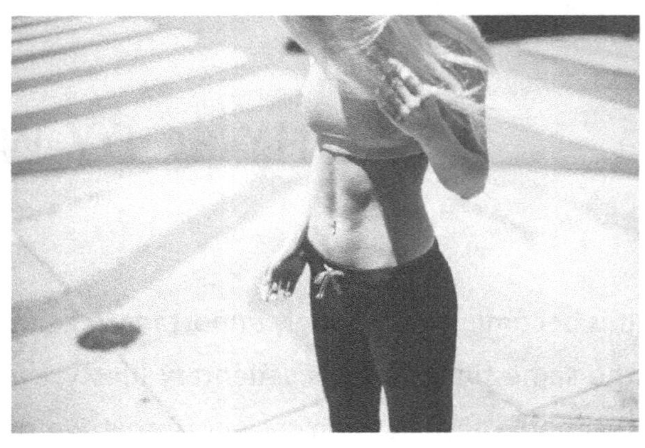 diabetes type 2, and chronic inflammatory diseases. Additionally, cancers have been associated with being overweight or obese. These include gallbladder, colon, breast, uterine, prostate, rectal, and ovarian cancers. Women and men can benefit from reducing the chances of acquiring the types of cancers predisposed to their sex.

A healthy heart is needed for proper growth and development. Poor heart health leads to failure to thrive. While at rest, the basal metabolic rate of an obese individual is higher than in individuals who have a healthy weight. The more the work the heart is expected to perform, the more the risk of getting a heart disease. If the artery supplying the heart muscle with blood gets blocked by things such as cholesterol due to obesity, you get a heart attack. A proper weight is ideal for longevity since you won't have to use drugs to address a failing heart of high blood pressure.

An extra weight means that you have to use more energy even for small activities. It becomes difficult to do healthful activities like exercises and eating healthy. The body needs more calories but it cannot burn the extra calories efficiently. The likelihood of hitting the gym reduces and the individual prefers to do activities that do not summon much of their efforts. This leads to a vicious cycle of weight gain and more health problems.

Overweight individuals are more likely to develop osteoarthritis from wear and tear of the cartilages lining the joint spaces. The extra weight put on the joints leads to more stress and shear forces. Maintaining a healthy body weight is important in preventing this type of arthritis. The joints will allow the individual to exercise and get healthier. Muscle sprains, strains, and sport-related injuries can also benefit from people who are flexible. Obese people who cut their weight by even a small percentage are less likely to suffer from gout.

A healthy weight is necessary for a properly functioning reproductive system. Obesity can lead to infertility and disturbances in the menstrual cycles in women. Many other systems are affected by weight problems. Snoring and difficulties in breathing such as asthma can result from excess fat in the tummy. Moreover, having a healthy weight gives one a good figure that fosters social relationships.

What is a Healthy Weight?

The body weight is made up of muscle, fat, bone, water, and any other compound found in the body. An unhealthy weight is a weight that comes mainly from too much fat. To accurately determine what causes the bulk of the weight of an individual may be a

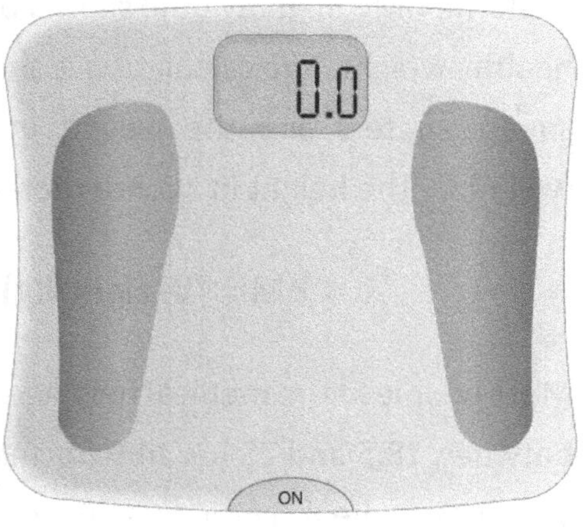

difficult or even impossible task. The commonly used parameters such as the weight-hip ratio and BMI have their advantages and disadvantages. The idea is to give the individual an approximate figure to work on while seeking to attain their healthy weight. As such, your ideal weight is bound to differ from that of others considering that there are many factors in play. The ideal healthy weight of an individual should put into context the age, sex, height, bone density, and fat-muscle ratio.

The BMI (Body Mass Index)

The body mass index is an estimate of how healthy an individual is compared to the rest of the population by use of weight and height. It assumes that the more the calculated figure, the unhealthier an individual is because of an excess of the fat deposits. This tool has been used to screen people and identify those individuals who are at an increased risk of heart diseases, diabetes, and even cancer. It is appropriate for people who are at least 20 years of age regardless of their sex. In essence, it can save one the trouble of doing more advanced tests to measure if they are healthy.

With the BMI, an individual should be able to achieve and maintain a healthy weight. The calculation is simple once you know the height in square meters and the weight in kilograms. Simply dividing the weight by the height in square meters gives the BMI.

$$BMI = [Weight(kg) \div height\ (m^2)]$$

Most people in the medical field agree that the normal BMI should be between 18.5 and 25 (or 24.9 for females). Having a BMI of less than 18.5 is not healthy since you are predisposed to problems with undernutrition. Anything above 25 in BMI is classified as excess weight. However, for purposes of distinguishing the risk groups, overweight individuals are those with a reading between 25 and 30 (29.9 for females). Obesity begins from a BMI of 30 onwards and it is further sub-classified;

- Class 1- BMI of between 30 and 35
- Class 2- BMI of 35 to 40
- Class 3- BMI of 40 or more.

The more obese you are (higher BMI), the more the chances that you will get some form of illness.

The biggest problem with using the BMI is estimating a weight problem is its inability to directly measure the total body fat content. Therefore, a person who has high-fat content for one reason or another may be falsely classified as healthy if they have a normal BMI. A big muscle mass of an individual can make one weigh heavier than a person who has more fat. Similarly, people who have muscle atrophy as in the geriatric population may be thought healthier when actually they have more fat. If BMI is used in children, it will not have the same meaning. This makes it impossible to use BMI across all ages. The body fat of kids differs across the age groups and sexes.

The Hip-Waist Ratio

Using the hip-waist ratios to screen for weight problems reveals more than the BMI. It gives a better clue about the ideal weight of the individual as well as the specific health risks. If this modality was used in place of BMI, it would capture more people who should address weight matters more seriously. The waist-hip ratio (WHR) is a measure of the waist circumference compared to that of the hip. To come up with the WHR, one needs to measure separately the circumferences of the hip and the waist. The hip is expected to be wider than the waist.

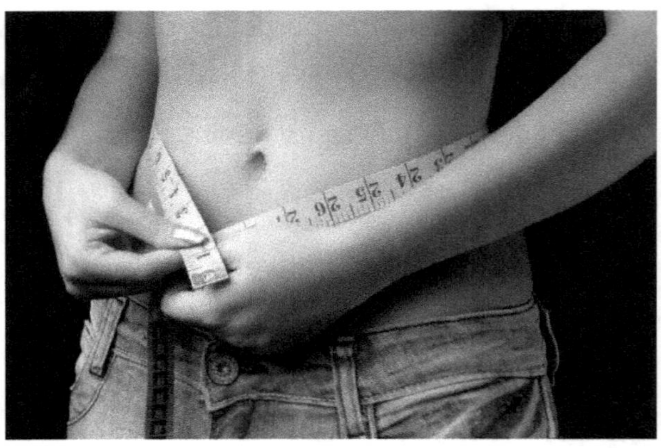

Dividing the waist by the hip circumference gives the WHR. A figure above 1 for males and 0.9 for females means that one has a high chance of acquiring one of the many heart or blood vessel diseases. 0.9-0.99 WHR of men and 0.8-0.89 WHR of females is associated with a lower risk of the heart health issues. Men with WHR of less than 0.9 as well as women whose WHR readings are below 0.8 are much less affected by cardiovascular adverse events. The lower the WHR, the healthier and reproductive the individual is.

WHR Norms			
	Healthy	Good	Average	Unhealthy
Female	<0.8	0.75-0.79	0.8-0.89	>0.9
Male	<0.9	0.85-0.89	0.9-0.99	>1

The most effective method is the use of both BMI and hip-waist ratio together. This will show the amount of fat deposited in your body and also its distribution patters.

Two people of one sex with the same height, weight, and hence BMI readings may have different WHRs. If one is apple shaped, more fat accumulates on the waist and they get a higher WHR. A pear-shaped individual will have a lower WHR because the fat deposition is concentrated in the hip area. The former individual is unhealthy while the latter is actually healthier. The downside of the WHR is that it still lacks the ability to identify the total fat percentage. However, it remains to be useful in health estimation because it can estimate some fat percentage in the body.

How to estimate your Basal Metabolic Rate

The basal metabolic rate (BMR) is simply the calorie burn that is required to run your body systems. Even without moving an inch, there is a significant amount of calories that your body uses to sustain the normal function of the body. The processes supported in the BMR include breathing, circulation, synthesis, and transport of enzymes and many other activities. All these processes are considered in the estimation of the BMR.

The BMR is closely related to the body metabolism. This means that a variation in the metabolism such as through changes in weight will lead to a change in the BMR. The BMR is an estimate of the 24-hour calorie requirement to stay alive. Through the BMR, you burn up as much as 60 % of the total daily calorie burn. This makes the knowledge of an individual's BMR very important in maintaining a healthy weight.

The BMR can be changed through some deliberate adjustments such as increasing the lean muscle mass. The factors that influence an individual's metabolism the most can lead to a significant change in the BMR. While identifying the exact factors that dictate your metabolism may be difficult, it would be useful to act on those factors when trying to lose weight.

To calculate the BMR, many attempts have been advanced to monitor the oxygen use and carbon dioxide elimination in subjects who have fasted for 12 hours while asleep. The analysis is almost accurate because oxygen is used up during metabolism and carbon dioxide is its product. This measurement is done in a laboratory under strict conditions that allow quantitative and qualitative studies on the gases of respiration. Formulas have been derived from the data and they have proved to be so accurate that they are considered effective and efficient in measuring the BMR.

In Mifflin St. Jeor's equation, the gender, weight, height, and age are used to come up with a mathematical estimate of the BMR. This online tool can help you get your BMR estimate.

The rates of metabolism are different across ages, gender, and height of subjects. The rate decreases with increasing age because of a decline in the muscle mass with advancing age. Women have lower BMRs than men because they have a lower ratio of muscle to fat. Additional factors that change the BMR are stress levels and disease states and they should be considered in the calculation where possible.

MOST EFFECTIVE METHODS OF FAT BURNING

Our diet program uses the most effective methods of fat burning. They are aimed at decreasing the total calories in the body and burning the residual excesses. Our fat burning recipe is made of detoxification, low carbohydrate intake, low-fat consumption, and intermittent fasting. When the body is free from toxins, it can concentrate on working for you to burn fat. However, we don't want to overwork the body and so we offer it a low-carb and a low fat diet. Intermittent fasting will deal with the rest of the calories even more effectively. They utilize the body's own pathways to achieve the aim of maintaining a healthy weight.

Detoxification

Our detoxification program aims to optimize the body's internal system. The liver is the chief detoxifying organ and it needs to function properly to eliminate excess fat cells. Fat tissues are useful to the body since they provide insulation, injury prevention, and energy when needed. On the other hand, excess fat cells that are overburdened tend to cause problems by inflammation since they are picked up by the immune system. It is important to keep a balance in the total body fat composition so as to get the benefits and not harm from these fat cells.

Proper fat metabolism depends on the liver function. Supporting and augmenting the function of the liver is an effective way to burn calories. The liver works to detoxify 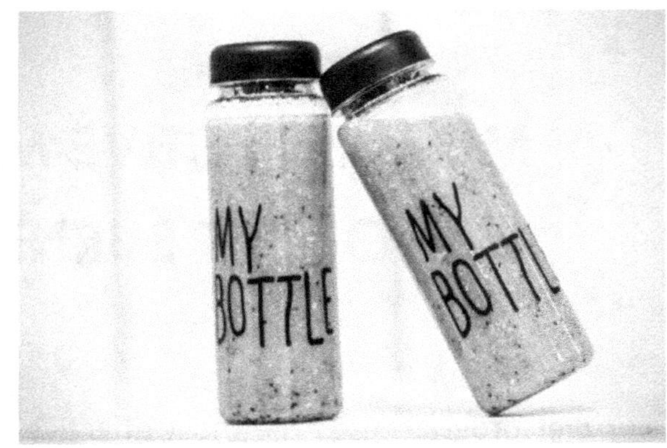 many substances from the diet. It also produces hormones and helps in digestion, temperature regulation, amongst many other critical functions. When the liver is working under normal conditions, it is tasked with the removal of fat from the blood. The liver cells can get overwhelmed by the fat and become fatty. Any injury to the liver leads to a fat metabolism problem since fat is not removed appropriately from the circulation. It ends up recycling in the liver through the hepatic portal vein.

The other reason why the liver burns excess calories is its ability to control the blood sugars. When you eat carbohydrates, the ultimate nutrient is glucose which is a source of instant energy to the body tissues. The liver can sense the need for glucose and mobilize the manufacturing units to produce more. It can also sense the presence of excess sugars in the blood and it will convert it to sugar stores known as glycogen. Both processes are vital for survival and they should be maintained in the optimum. If the liver does not function well, it will have problems with breaking down the stored sugar energy. Insulin, the hormone of abundance will instruct the liver to store more. Liver congestion leads to excess storage with less breakdown leading to obesity.

Detoxifying the liver helps to burn more calories since it is good for liver health. Toxins tend to build up in fat tissues when the liver is congested. The body won't burn the toxin-high fat cells and excess fat remains in the body. This worsens the condition because more fat means more toxin stores. The individual feels tired and sluggish, hence unable to perform healthful habits like exercising. Detoxification ensures that toxins are flushed away from the system making the liver and other organs function as expected. A healthy body is efficient in eliminating calories which are not needed.

Low Carb Consumption

Carbohydrates from starchy foods end up being deposited in the body. Eating a low carb diet increases your chances of cutting weight healthily. The main source of fuel in the body is carbohydrates and many cells prefer it to other sources of energy such as fat. After ingestion, starch is broken down to simple sugars and eventually to glucose mainly. When glucose is absorbed into the bloodstream, it causes a surge in the blood glucose levels. Hormones such as insulin and growth hormone are stimulated to store and utilize the glucose.

There are many types of carbohydrate sources and most food processors use it to add taste and flavor. Naturally produced sugars are better than their processed counterparts. The mechanism of action that leads to calorie burning in a low carb diet is storing less. Natural sugars are slowly metabolized and broken down into the active sugars. The amount of glucose that enters the blood when one eats natural sugar is reduced when compared to refined sugars. A low carb diet should provide just the needed amount of sugar without causing excess deposition. The lowered intake of carbohydrates in the diet leads to less insulin secretion and reduced storage.

Reducing the calories consumed from carbs by 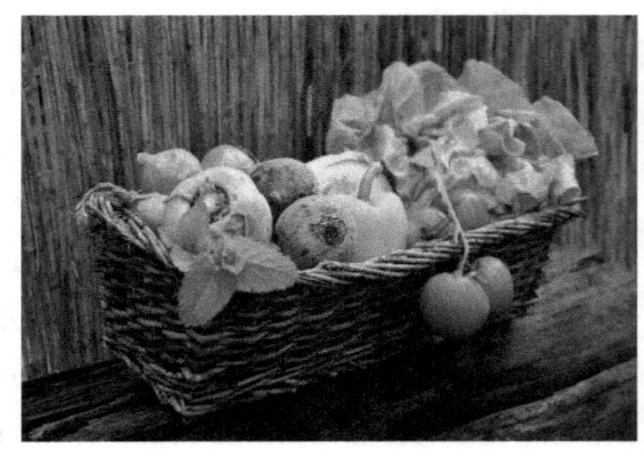 at least 500 can help one lose 1 pound or more per week. Further restriction leads to further weight loss especially if it is coupled with exercise or other weight intervention tools. The low carb diet also prevents diabetes, hypertension, cardiovascular disease, and associated complications such as the metabolic syndrome. A diet plan can be the only way to reduce the risk of diseases and cancers since it works to prevent the introduction of excess toxins in the body. Weight gain is reversible through simple dietary changes. A moderately low carbohydrate intake is that which involves eating less than 130 grams of carbs per day. Low carb diets should ensure that the carb intake is between 50 and 130 grams per day. A more restrictive diet can achieve a very low carb intake if the individual takes no more than a total of 50 grams of carbs per day.

The advantage of doing the low carb diet is that an individual can eat the other types of foods normally and will still lose weight. Even the carbs need not be overly restricted to get the weight cut. As long as you avoid the likes of potatoes, refined sugars, and wheat products which are loaded with high carb levels, you can get a good weight control with eating the rest of the carbohydrates. There are many options to choose from in low carbohydrate food intake. One is allowed to eat meat, eggs, veggies, cheese, and other sources of low carbs in the diet.

Low Fat Consumption

Low fat intake can help one not only lose but also maintain weight. Fatty foods have much higher calories than most other types of foods. Reducing the fat consumption and replacing the diet with alternative foods with fewer fats helps in cutting weight. Some types of fats have been implicated in causing obesity while some fatty foods are actually beneficial. While aiming at cutting the daily fat intake, the individual should ensure that the high-fat containing products are stuck off the diet. They can be replaced with those that contain some fat and are healthful.

Saturated fats found in meat, lard, and butter contributes to a great percentage of fat in the diet. These should be avoided to help mitigate weight problems. Trans fats are processed fat from plant vegetables and they are unhealthy. They add to weight problems as well as general health issues. Unsaturated fats such as those from sunflower oil, corn oil, olive oil, rapeseed oil, and omega 3 fatty acids are better for healthy living. They may contain high calories just like saturated fats and caution must be exercised when using them if an individual wants to lose weight.

Just like carbs, fats are absorbed into the body and stored for times of starvation. When an individual is on the verge of starvation, the body shifts to make the necessary arrangements to sustain the person for as long as possible. Fatty foods frequent in the diet will be stored in the body in preparation for lean times. Reducing the fat intake in the diet means that the amount of fat available for storage is reduced. The rest of the fat is used up and very little is stored. During starvation, fat is only required when the body is sure that it has exhausted the carbohydrate stores. Unless the period of starvation continues for long, the body may not even need the fat since the liver will break down its glucose.

Whether you take fewer carbs or fats, you will ultimately have a reduced weight. The point is to reduce the total caloric intake which is balanced off by the energy expenditure. Similar food intakes for carbs and fats are effective in ensuring that an individual loses weight. Reducing these types of nutrients in the diet and supplementing with proteins promotes healthy weight loss. The high protein, low carb, and low-fat foods offer satiety with decreased calorie intake. Since the body must burn calories for energy production, more calories utilized versus that which is ingested lead to a weight loss. Fiber foods which are free from carbs and fats increase fullness and you won't eat frequently.

When an individual chooses to lose weight using the diet, the main challenge is fighting cravings. Food cravings are a serious cause of regaining weight. However, an individual who eats low carbs or low fats can manage the cravings better than those who stick to stricter diets. The quality of the food taken is just as important as the food choice itself. Some junk foods having added sugars may offer the promise of a healthy fat-free diet option.

Intermittent Fasting

Many people underestimate the power of fasting in weight loss yet it is common knowledge that it leads to a reduced caloric intake. Starvation is lack of food for one reason or another and it should not be confused with fasting which is voluntary. Intermittent fasting (IF) is the deliberate withholding of food for a period after which an individual eats normally. Staying without food can be a daunting task for the beginner but with time it becomes easy to cope. Strictly looking at IF, the individual lives by changing the cycle and pattern of eating.

Almost everybody fasts at night when they are sleeping. Intermittent fasting is, therefore, an elongation of the normal physiology of fasting to achieve health benefits such as loss of weight. Fasting, which is technically any

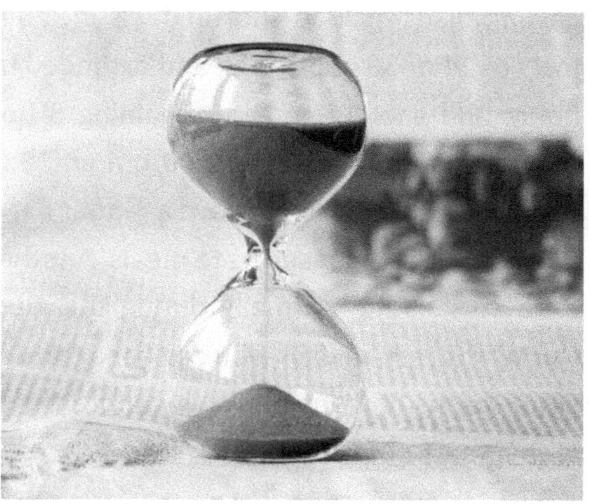

time one is not eating, gives the body a break from absorption and storage of nutrients. The time becomes a period of burning excess calories which is necessary to maintain the metabolic processes. Usually, the body will first use all the calories found in the bloodstream before shifting to other sources. After using up the instant sources of energy, the liver produces some more energy from burning the carb stores and then the fat stores. The body will slowly shift to use of fats in what is called ketogenic metabolism where fat is broken down to form ketones.

Surprisingly, the energy powerhouse from glycogen stores can last for up to 36 hours although it can be depleted earlier. After a period of fasting for about 24 hours, the body will have no choice but to get energy from ketones. The fat stores in peripheral tissues are seemingly unlimited but are not easily accessible. It takes some period of fasting to finally get to burn the fat stored in the subcutaneous tissues. Fasting even for a few hours has significant weight benefits for the individual. Shorter fasts are better because they can be done more often without much straining.

Fasting plans include shorter fasts including the 16:8, 20:4; longer fasts of 24 or 36 hours, 5:2; and extended fasting. You can fast for 16 hours and eat during the remaining 8 hours daily. An example is eating anytime between 12:00 pm and 8:00 pm. Alternatively, you can do a 20 hour fast and have a 4-hour period of eating a large heavy meal or two smaller separate meals. Another way of fasting is to have 5 days of eating normally during the week and two fasting days. During the fasting days, you can eat a total of fewer than 500 calories. Other forms of fasting involving more than 48 hours are occasioned with nutrient deficiencies.

The best way to achieve the calorie burning fasting methods is, to begin with, a short duration plan and advance slowly. Abrupt withdrawal of your eating pattern in the extremes may be unhealthy. Your body needs to get used to staying without food for more hours first before you take on a 2-day fast design. Making a routine in which food schedules are put father apart can be the first step for guaranteed success.

A combination of detox, low carbs, and low fats in the diet together with occasional intermittent fasting is a very effective and healthy weight loss tool. The total calories in the body will be dramatically reduced and the remaining will be burned effectively. A good liver allows you to fast for even longer because it is competent in commanding gluconeogenesis.

TYPES AND BENEFITS OF NUTRITION

Eating healthy begins with knowing the types of nutrition that are needed by the body. Nutrients are the vital materials that are required to sustain life. Failure to provide adequate nutrients to the body cells leads to a myriad of preventable health problems. Consequently, overprovision of one type of nutrient at the expense of the others leads to disease states.

In general, the essential nutrients are classified as macronutrients or micronutrients depending on the amount which must be found in the diet to maintain normal growth and development of cells. Vitamins and minerals are therefore classified as micronutrients while proteins, carbohydrates, and fat make much of the macronutrients in food. The other types of nutrients include water which is extremely essential and forms as much as 60% of the body weight and roughage. Since we need fibre or roughage and water in large amounts, they are considered as part of the macronutrients.

Foods are also classified according to their major input in metabolism. For instance, energy giving foods are those which have a lot of fat and carbs. They provide a lot of energy for almost all types of activities running inside the body. Protective foods are those which are predominantly vitamins or minerals and they help boost the immunity amongst other protective roles. Proteins are referred to as growing foods because they are the building structures of the body.

The foods we eat usually contain a mixture of nutrients. For convenience, the foods are grouped as carbs, fats, proteins, or vitamins according to the type of nutritious content that is found in greater amounts within the food. The amount of calories provided by the food type varies across the food species and is influenced by many factors including preparation and processing. However, it is expected that a gram of carbohydrate or protein will have fewer calories (4 calories) than a gram of fatty food (9 calories).

Carbohydrates

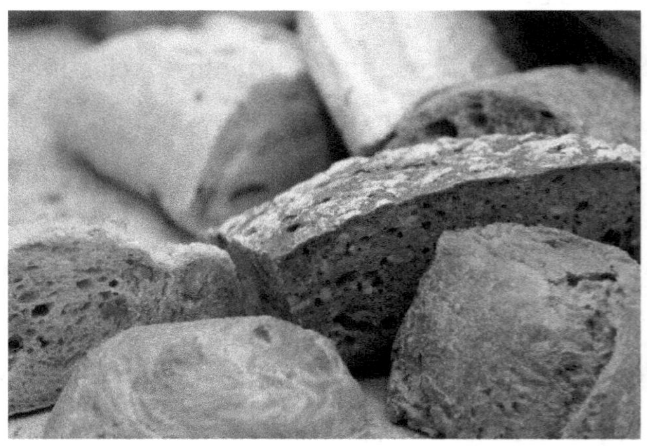

Carbohydrates are synonymous with sugar because that is the common thing about all carb sources. The number and availability of the sugars vary such that carbs are further classified into monosaccharides, disaccharides, or polysaccharides. The subclassification is relevant in some groups of people such as those suffering from diabetes. People with diabetes should avoid too many simple carbohydrates (monosaccharides and disaccharides) since they tend to worsen the high levels of glucose in the blood. You can get simple sugars from eating honey, sugar cane, sweet fruits, biscuits, and sugar. Complex sugars are derived from starch and cellulose.

Carbohydrates are the main fuel source for the body. Organ systems cannot function properly without energy. The brain, heart, kidney, musculoskeletal system, and nervous system require good amounts of carbs to be optimized. Excess carbohydrates are stored in the liver and muscle tissue for future use. Carbs can help protect against disease by modulating the immune system. Antigens presented to the white blood cells are made up of carbs joined to proteins. The presence of an adequate amount of carbs in the body spares proteins and fats from being converted to sources of energy.

Healthy sources of carbs include whole grains, beans, veggies, and fruits. Whole grain sources of high carb content include barley, brown rice, oatmeal, quinoa, and whole grain breakfast cereals. Melons, apples, pears, bananas, and berries are great fruit sources of carbs. Starchy vegetables are peas, carrots, sweet potatoes, and yams. Legumes such as lentils, black beans, and soybeans are recommendable sources of carbs. Low-fat milk and some types of yogurts also provide adequate amounts of carbs. Low carb food sources are non-starchy vegetables such as spinach, cabbage, tomatoes, and mushrooms. Nuts, seeds, soy milk, and tofu can be taken by people who don't need too much carb contents in their diet.

Fibre

Fibre is part of the carbohydrates that are not digested. They pass through the gut and help in bulk-forming. Sources of fibre include carrots, bananas, peas, beans, whole grains, cabbages, and cassava. Fibre helps in satiety and reduces the calories taken in the diet. It prevents and manages constipation through making the stool soft and bulky. Fibre also ensures a slow and steady release of nutrients in the gut.

Proteins

Proteins build every cell of the body and should be considered in the diet. They are used for growth, repair or damaged tissue and maintenance of body processes. Antibodies to fight pathogens; hormones for mood regulation and growth; and other substances such as albumin and parts of the red blood cells are all made from proteins. Proteins are not supposed to be used to provide fuel unless the need arises as in starvation.

Amino acids are the basic units of the protein chains. Some of the amino acids are synthesized by the body. Those which cannot be synthesized must be sourced from the diet. Healthy sources of proteins include white meat and fish. Eggs are known for providing many essential amino acids in the body. The other great sources of proteins are soy, nuts, lentils, milk, beans, and some types of grains. Animal sources of proteins are better than plant sources.

Fats

Fats have the reputation of being rich in calories and energy. They are especially useful in young children who need high amounts of energy to sustain both their metabolism and playing. Fats and oils make food tastier and fulfilling. They can either be saturated or unsaturated depending on the state in a cool environment. Saturated fats are solid at low temperatures while unsaturated fats remain in liquid form at a similar temperature.

Unsaturated fats are healthful and can be sourced from fish, oil seeds like sunflower, maize, and groundnut oils. Unlike proteins, plant sources of fats and oils are healthier than animal sources. Other foods that are excellent in providing fat in the diet are milk products, avocado, and meat products. The benefits of good fats include the balance of blood glucose and reducing the incidences of type 2 diabetes, and heart disease. They are potent anti-inflammatory agents that protect the individual from cancers, arthritis, and Alzheimer's disease.

Vitamins

Vitamins are useful in protecting the body from disease. They include vitamins A, B complex, C, and D. eating vitamins ensures that you have good vision, 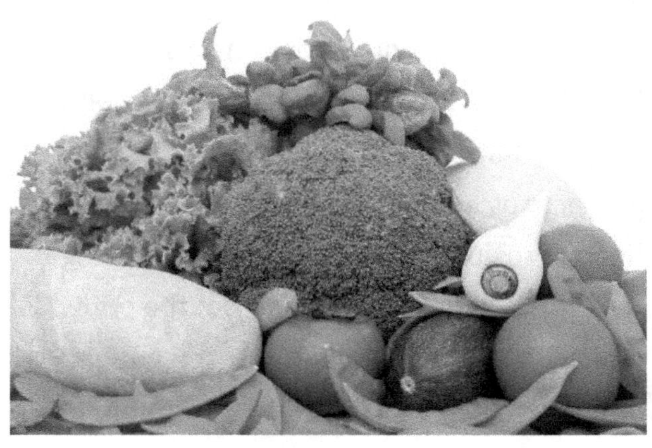 skin, and bone health. Fat-soluble vitamins A, D, E, and K dissolve in fats and are insoluble in water. They are only utilizable if fat is present. The rest of the vitamins are water soluble and because of this property, cannot be stored in the body tissues. The vitamins may protect from some types of cancers since they are anti-oxidants in nature. Wound healing and immune boost are ensured by vitamins. Good sources of vitamins include vegetables, fruits, and bacteria from the intestines.

Minerals

Calcium, magnesium, phosphorus, zinc, iron, and copper are some examples of minerals that are required for proper functioning of the body. Zinc boosts the immunity and helps in healing of excoriations. Iron is vital for production, function, and survival of the red blood cells. Calcium and magnesium help in maintaining the normal blood pressure and muscle function. Milk, cheese, dairy, meat, eggs, vegetables, table salt, and water are sources of minerals.

Water

Water is one of the most important nutrients in the body that is necessary for life. It cools the system, baths the cells, supplies nutrients to the cells and tissues, and acts as a lubricating fluid allowing the heart and lungs to move freely. Drinking water aids in flushing toxins from the body. It also prevents constipation in the gut and improves the motility and absorption of food contents. Water sources include fluids 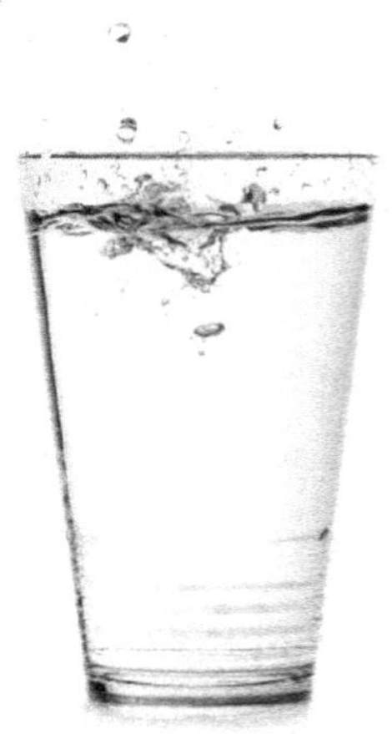 that you take as drinks and plant sources such as fleshy fruits and vegetables. It is difficult to monitor the exact amount of fluid that an individual should take. However, the color of urine and feeling of thirst are reliable markers of water in the body.

GETTING READY FOR
A HEALTHY DIET

Weight loss will need one to change their lifestyle and it needs adequate preparation. You need to know what to expect and set goals to achieve over time. A transition from unhealthy habits to healthy alternatives is necessary. You should practice keeping a routine of when to wake up; what to eat; when to sleep; how long you should sleep; and so on and so forth. This helps in maintaining the new healthful habits. You won't have to struggle with the health choices if you know what you are expected to achieve every day.

Setting a Goal

To decide how much you should lose in the quest for weight loss, you need a goal. The goal can be derived from the weight calculation using either the BMI or the WHZ or even both. Setting a realistic goal is as good as achieving it. The baseline weight measurement is a point of reference for gauging your progress. You can choose to hit any weight within the normal BMI range. Weekly weight loss targets can be set and then re-evaluated at the end of the period. Some people prefer to look at it in the long run and they will set targets spanning longer periods of weeks to months. Photos of your current figure can also help in setting the goal. It can be a source of motivation if you can consistently achieve your set targets.

Motivating Yourself

People drop out of the weight programs because they lack enough motivation. Motivation can make all the difference especially when there seems to be no progress. 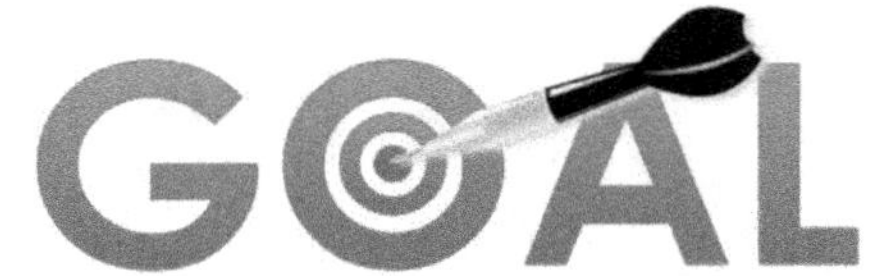 Such a state of a plateau phase is discouraging because an individual would wish to always see a progress at every weight measurement. Motivation becomes a crucial ingredient to success in weight loss. Friends and family members can motivate and encourage you from time to time. However, you need to foster your internal sources of motivation which actually tend to be stronger and more effective in long-term goals. Always maintain a positive perspective and expect better results in the future. Find a supporting community which can help you both psychologically and physically. It may be a wrong move in your exercise that is holding you back from hitting the target. For more on motivation, use the motivation book. It has details on how to go about different difficult scenarios in weight loss.

Remove all Unhealthy Foods

The environment has an impact on your lifestyle choices. The food stored in your kitchen can make you eat healthy or unhealthy. For proper weight loss, you have to remove all the temptations of eating sweet, sugary, and fatty foods which are high in calories. Remove all the junk food from the refrigerator. Clean the entire house of junk foods also so that you don't live with the temptation to satisfy your cravings. You are likely to eat what's in the refrigerator when you are idle because it does not require much preparation. It may seem like a waste but you will realize how much profit it earns when you lose weight. You should be in a position to distinguish the bad foods from the good ones. Whenever you are in doubt, you can create another category of foods in the refrigerator as those which you are not sure about. Once you have sorted them, use resources such as the internet to identify the value of the foodstuffs. For instance, if you want to eat nuts, you should be careful not to eat groundnuts since they are actually legumes and not nuts.

Stop Unhealthy Snacking

There are many reasons why one would opt for a sugary snack. Stress can lower an individual's moods and they will want to eat something that will lighten up

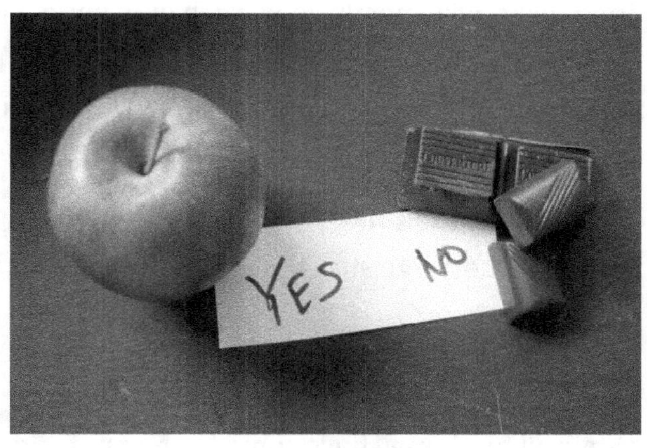

their smile. This is usually a snack that is sweet to the tongue. While it may work to elevate your moods, it is not a healthy diet choice. Other people eat snacks at lunch to give them a rush of energy to push them through the day. They are convenient for many who don't have the time to prepare a healthy meal during the lunch breaks. Getting used to unhealthy snacking may lead to regaining weight even with intense workouts. The body only needs some energy from the food. The rest of the calories will end up being stored for future purposes. If you keep taking sugary snacks and drinks, you will end up increasing the total calorie intake. If you must take something outside meal times, insist on a fruit or a vegetable. They have good amounts of sugars enough to supply you with instant energy. Moreover, they are natural sources of healthy calories.

Don't Eat From Restaurants

Restaurants make it difficult to eat healthily. It is an environment of many unhealthy options for junk foods. You can do better in weight loss if you decide to eat at home where you prepare good food. The cooking at home ideology helps one to appreciate the process that healthy food needs to pass through before you can eat. Fast and quick food fixes will mostly lead to high-calorie intake unless one has carefully chosen the right type of foods. If you have set your kitchen into a hub of low-calorie foods, there is should be no reason why you will end up cooking unhealthy food. At home, you have many options and you won't decide on a high-calorie menu for lack of a variety. This is why it is better to stick to eating at the comfort of home at all times.

Avoid Consuming Empty Calories

While all foods may have some form of nutrition, empty calorie foods are those which add a supply of energy without a reasonable amount of nutrition. These foods must be avoided since they lead to weight problems. The following foods are considered empty calories- they are processed with a lot of fat or sugar:

- ☐ *Ice cream*
- ☐ *Biscuits*
- ☐ *Pastries*

- ☐ *Sweetened fruit drinks*
- ☐ *Soda*
- ☐ *Sausage*
- ☐ *Bacon*
- ☐ *Hot dogs*
- ☐ *Pizza*
- ☐ *Burgers*
- ☐ *Candy*

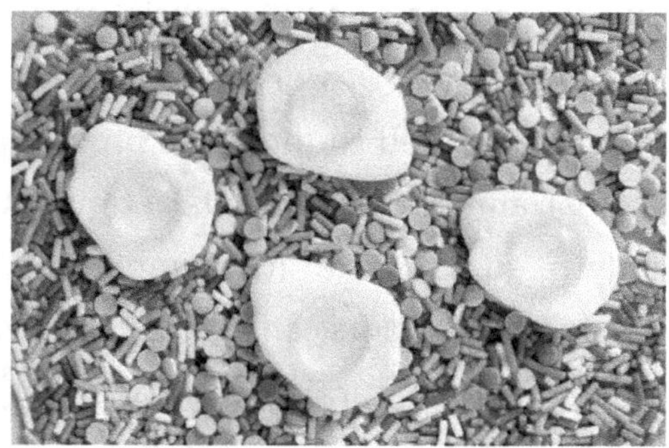

Stop Artificial Beverages, Alcohol, and Smoking

Alcohol and other beverages are sources of high calories and are almost devoid of good nutrients. The problem with alcohol and beverage drinking is that one gets addicted and it becomes difficult to quit cold turkey. The body gets used to the stimulant or tranquilizing effects of the drinks and one can't physically or psychologically tolerate a withdrawal. Tobacco smoking is a harmful habit that is equally addictive and leads to breathing problems and cancers. Tobacco has been associated with weight problems and it should be avoided in individuals who want to cut their weights. There are friendly beverages such as the green herbal tea which can replace the other types of unhealthy beverages. All efforts to stop the consumption of alcohol should be put in place since the benefits in weight loss are tremendous. People addicted to nicotine can have chewing gums or nicotine patches as a replacement.

Use Artificial Sweeteners and Honey

Tooth decay is caused by an activity of bacteria working on sugars in your teeth. The bacteria feed on sugars to grow in their colonies. To prevent this, you need to replace your table sugar with artificial sweeteners or honey. Artificial sweeteners have the reputation of having low calories and at the same time provide a sweeter taste when compared to the same amount of the commonly used sugars. A small amount is hundreds of times sweeter to the tongue and you'll only need to use a little amount to taste. Pure honey if taken in moderate amounts can actually help one boost their immune system. Since it is a natural source of sugar, it has nutritious amounts of vitamins B, A, C, D, E, and K. Its mineral content of magnesium, iron, calcium, potassium, sodium, and many other minerals are of great use to the body.

Have an Abundance of Healthy Foods

In preparing to live healthily and shed some more weight, make it a point to always have a stock of fruits and vegetables. You can have the willpower to cut the weight but if you don't have the plan and the skill power, you are likely to fail. To avoid excuses, shop for enough fruits and veggies and stock them in your kitchen. It would be great to do a weekly stop-over at the local grocery and make sure that you pick enough greens for the diet. Store the food in the fridge so that you are surrounded by good foods at all times. The temptation to eat unhealthy foods comes and becomes strong when you don't have an option of healthy foods. Be sure to remove any doubts by working with a food schedule that will instruct on the type of foods to buy to last a week.

To-Do List

People can forget things and remember them later when it is of no use to them. In weight loss programs, it is important to be consistent in practicing healthful habits. Skipping a day could make one lag behind for a long time and find it hard to recover the lost gains. In a busy schedule, you are more prone to forgetfulness as 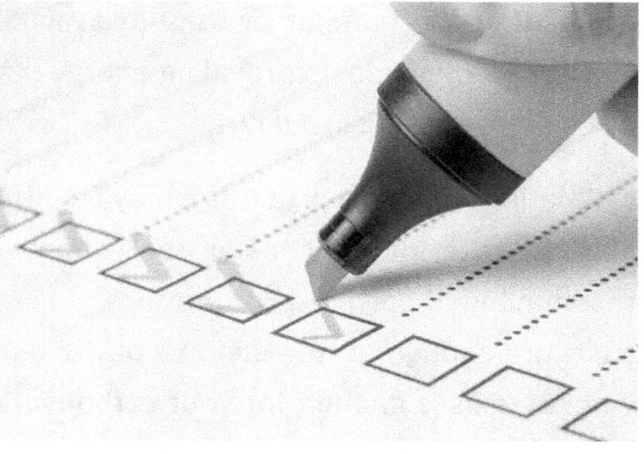 you try to decongest the brain's memory by doing only what you consider as significant. You can forget to use the stairs when going to your office. To avoid all the inconveniences caused by a congested memory, you can hang a to-do list on the fridge or a place that you are sure to pass by the first thing when you wake up. This will act as a reminder to help you do all things routinely without missing anything. Once you accomplish a task, mark it as complete and then go for the next task.

Regular Small Meals

We need to eat to survive, grow, and develop normally. Food is not the problem in weight gain but rather, the amount of calories taken causes us problems. Eating regular small volumes of foods makes it better to control weight.

A frequency of 5 times a day of eating 3 meals and 2 snacks is the best way to ensure that we get only what we need for energy and metabolic processes. A large single meal a day may lead to overeating as one tries to compensate for the body's energy expenditure. Additionally, lesser meal frequencies tend to be full of the temptations to eat high-carb or sugary foods. The 3 meals a day plan can reduce the number of calories available for storing per meal. Snacks will be useful in providing energy between meals and should not be more than 2 in a day.

Estimating the right portion size may be difficult. Use anything handy like the size of your palm to estimate the size of the daily recommended portions. For instance, 5 hand fulls of vegetables and fruits are enough for the diet in a day. 6 ounces of grains preferably whole grains is enough for your carbohydrate needs. You can do 5 half-ounces of proteins and about 6 teaspoonfuls of oil per day. Don't eat until the stomach is 100% full; stop eating when you feel 80% full. This will need some practice before mastering the amount of portion that one needs for the day. Men have a slightly higher BMR than women and they can eat one measure more than women.

A Sample Serving Size per BMI				
	Vegetables & fruits	Fats	Carbs	Proteins
Men (BMR 24 calories/kg	5 servings	6 teaspoonfuls	6 Oz whole grain	5 Oz beans, meat e.t.c.
Women (BMR 23 calories/ kg)	4 servings	5 teaspoonfuls	5 Oz whole grains	4 Oz beans, meat e.t.c.

Tips:

- [ ] *Read the food labels*
- [ ] *Learn more about food types and their nutrition*
- [ ] *Some food preparations have higher calories when processed*
- [ ] *You may add an extra serving if you will be performing high intensity duties or workouts*

Eat At least 2 Hours Before You Go To Bed

Sleep hygiene matters in weight loss. If you sleep immediately after a large dinner, you will have digestion problems, sleep irregularly, and gain weight in the long run. The dinner time should be adjusted accordingly to fit your sleeping program. If you must sleep at 10:00 pm, then the meal should be ready earlier and you should complete eating by 8:00 pm. The remaining time can be used to do something constructive. You need to avoid too much activity before bedtime since it will interfere with your sleep. Too much excitement before bedtime delays sleep. Similarly, lights from your smartphone can deter sleep. Choose to do things that won't require too much attention or energy after dinner. Poor bedtime habits will make you get to bed early but wake up feeling tired.

Wake Up Early

The earlier you wake up, the better position you will be to handle the day. You need to be organized and planned so that everything is done in its time. Waking up late will lead to either a postponing of an activity or skipping it altogether. An individual who wakes up early is more likely to have all the time to prepare a healthy breakfast or jog before going to work. This makes early waking a crucial part of salvaging issues with time management. To wake up early,

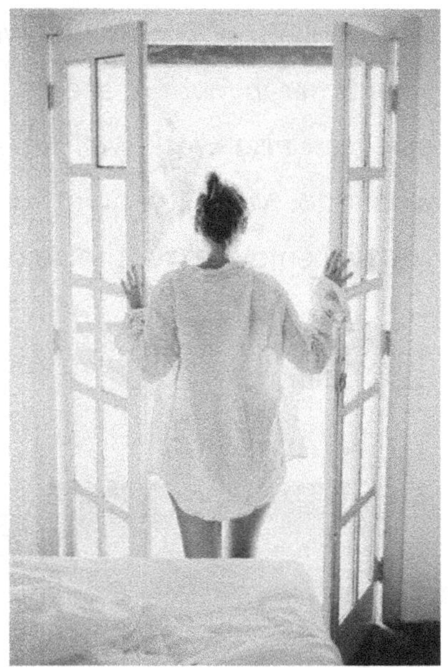

you'll need to sleep early and have adequate sleep in the bed. This involves a lot of discipline and training so that you have enough rest every day. Waking up early should not be done while sacrificing on the sleep time.

Have 8 Hours of Sleep

Sleep is the only time when the whole body rests. The brain, the nervous system, the musculature, the gut, and all other systems need to rest. You can't effectively light the gym weights if you didn't get enough sleep the previous night. The muscles will get fatigued and you will get cramps and other abnormalities. The digestive system needs time to digest the food contents eaten throughout the day. Without a balance of the hormones and a well-functioning nervous system, conduction problems will slow you down. A slow metabolism leads to weight gain since metabolic processes demand energy leading to the breakdown of calories. Do not let anything disturb the 8-hour sleep portion which you need to function well. You can use aromatherapy where scents induce your desire to sleep. A relaxing bath can also work well for sleep problems just as chamomile tea would do. Make it a point to get a good night's sleep every day and you will enjoy better the next day.

THE COMMON MISTAKES OF DIETING

Dieting is not free from challenges. Common mistakes may lead to undesirable results even with maximum effort to stay healthy. Some people do not realize the impact that these mistakes have on the program. One can get discouraged and quit the dieting plan because of these avoidable mistakes.

Monotony

In the desire to get maximum gains in a short time interval, people make the mistake of being too strict on the diet. The results may be encouraging at first when one loses a significant weight after a few weeks of dieting. However, the long-term survival is hindered by monotonous fruit and veggies in the diet. The diets lack enough nutrients to sustain the energy needs and the buildup of muscles. The dieter gets easy fatigability, which becomes a reason for quitting. It is important to be creative when one starts dieting and include a variety of foods in the diet.

Taking too little Calories

Some diet plans encourage reducing the amount of food intake to reduce the calories in the body. However, some people who may not know the exact number of calorie to take per day end up undernourished. The body metabolism may maladapt to the small amounts of food. The better way to approach reducing the calorie intake is to eat small but frequent meals with an interval of about 4 hours.

Dieting for no Clear Reason

People who are not resolute about why they are dieting will end up being discouraged when they don't achieve their targets. Before one begins the dieting plan, it is wise to assess the feasibility of the plan and have a reason to push you through hard moments in the program. When plateaus come, those who began the program with a definite reason will persevere.

Pushing too hard

Change must be approached in steps if it is expected to last. Taking too many items in a program at once may be overwhelming. Some dieters push themselves to the limit too soon even before their bodies get used to the new lifestyle. It is better to focus on simple milestones and take on one habit at a time. As the body adjusts, you can take on more with much ease.

Obsession with Leftovers

It is understandable when one gets obsessed with waste food. The thought of throwing away food makes one feel that they are wasting on resources. However, in dieting, being so much concerned with leftovers will lead to over-eating. The excess calories from the leftovers are often not counted as part of the total calorie intake. The dieter may find it difficult to cut and maintain weight when they seem to be doing everything right.

Lack of Portion Control

As one gets to choose healthy foods, the portion size matters. You may end up taking in too many calories while eating healthy food. Handfuls of healthy foods can load up more calories than unhealthy foodstuffs. It is necessary to practice portion size control in every bite during dieting to stay in shape.

PHASE 1:
DETOXIFYING & BOOSTING

After everything is set and you are ready to leave healthy, phase one of the journey is to detox and boost. The system has a maximum capacity of functioning and it can be reduced by toxins from food or drinks. Some dietary changes will serve to protect you from harmful toxins which have their way into the system. You may need a full week of daily detoxing and boosting to achieve maximum benefits. Essentially, the natural detox done by the liver and other organs such as the kidney and the skin is boosted. Once they are in good working condition, they favor weight loss and dieting programs.

The guidelines for the detoxifying and boosting phase comprise the phase 1 of the weight loss program. This initial phase lasts 7 days of intense cleansing of the body from toxic substances and increasing the circulation.

Phase 1 length = 7 days

You will stick to the healthy dietary changes mentioned above as you detox. This induction phase does not stress on being strict on the diet. You will need to first optimize the metabolism. Anyhow maintaining the correct balance of macronutrients is necessary and will be as follows;

Carbs : Proteins : Fats = 2 : 4 : 1

The caloric intake in this phase will be;

**Maximum calorie intake = 1200 calories
for women /1500 calories for men.**

This is because you don't want to get a sudden change in the dietary habits by limiting the calorie intake too much. However, you shouldn't also overburden the body with extra calories. Sticking to the recommended caloric intake will be necessary.

Boosting the Dormant Metabolism

The metabolism can be slowed down by disease processes and they make the individual slow in going about their daily activities. You may begin getting forgetful and having slow cognition if your body is full of toxins. The gut can't digest food as quickly as it should and you end up having less energy from the dietary intake. This may come despite an effort to take in more food. The problem is with the metabolism and it needs to be corrected so that the individual systems can function properly. Simple elimination of toxins using home-made detox remedies raises your metabolism to the appropriate range. Exercising gives you both a boost in metabolism and helps in detoxifying the system. As you workout, the skin sheds off toxic substances through sweating. The lungs work harder to drive out the excess buildup of lactic acid in the muscles. This leads to an increase in the metabolic rate where more oxygen is delivered to the tissues to support the rising demands.

Flush Away Toxins

Herbs and fruits that are taken in detox help cleanse the body. Toxins that build up in normal metabolism need to be channeled out of the body. Usually, there are systems in place to ensure that the toxins are taken care off as they get into the system. However, times come when the toxins build up and overwhelm the normal processes of excretion. This situation requires an external assistance from detox foods and juices to flush away toxic metabolites. The less the harmful substances, the less work the body has to do to detoxify. Therefore, detox helps optimize the body function of the various organs. More work can be done in anabolism and in support of the rest of the processes that go on in the nervous or cardiovascular systems. To achieve this desirable toxin-free state, one has to reduce and eventually eliminate the toxic foods that they eat. Eating the right foodstuffs that provide fiber, vitamins, minerals, and phytochemicals favor the metabolism.

Enhancing the Circulation

The two major circuits that conduct fluid in the body are the blood vessels and the lymphatic vessels. Blood and lymph interact to remove toxins from the body safely. It is important to have a well-working circulatory system which will lead to an increase in the rate of toxin removal. Exercises such as yoga and aerobics increase the blood flow in the system. When blood flows faster, it delivers nutrients faster and removes toxic metabolites faster. The blood from the arteries ends up in the capillaries which joint up to form veins. As blood flows towards the veins, some of it remains to form lymph which later rejoins the circulation. A boost in one circulatory circuit will work to boost the other circuit and the end result is a better function of the system.

Massage, sauna, and heat therapies help in improving the circulation of the blood. Mechanical compression of the muscles constricts the vessels and pushes blood back to the heart. Water therapy has been used to stimulate the lymphatic system to perform better detox functions. An aromatic bath is not only relaxing but it is also a way to improve the metabolism. Some therapies involve an alteration of hot and cold to boost the circulation. Warmth relaxes the vessels under the skin and cold makes them constrict. An alternation between warm and cold water in the shower behaves like a mechanical pump that acts on the blood vessels.

Part of the cleaning procedure involves drinking water. A lot of water is required during the initial phase of detox and boosting to dilute toxins. This makes it easier for the body to eliminate the toxic metabolites without causing harm to the organs. Sugary and junk foods deposit chemicals from preservatives in the body. They need to be eliminated from the diet and the toxins removed before one advances to the next phase. You can never go wrong with drinking a lot of water especially when you are thirsty. You will simply be replacing the water lost through breathing and sweating.

Chlorophyll Water

Chlorophyll is the green pigment that gives plants their color. Without chlorophyll, plants cannot survive. It can be rightly stated that this pigment is analogous to the blood which is the lifeline of human beings. Studies have shown that chlorophyll is very identical to hemoglobin which gives blood its function of carrying oxygen and carbon dioxide. The minor difference between the two structures is found in the core mineral compound. Hemoglobin has iron while chlorophyll has magnesium and that is the only biggest difference between the two minerals. It is no wonder that they are vital for the species that contain them.

Drawing the illustration that hemoglobin and chlorophyll have similar functions, we can get the benefits of chlorophyll pigment in our body systems. This green pigment helps in making our own hemoglobin and hence replenishing the red cell reserves. Drinking chlorophyll water helps boost the individual's well being and energy levels. That is why green foods are very healthful and should be part of every diet that aims at longevity. The pigment helps also in boosting one's immunity, maintaining skin health, and fighting inflammatory products.

Detoxing is necessary for people who want to lose weight and they can benefit from multiple lines of detoxification. This includes the use of chlorophyll water. The high levels of vitamins such as vitamin A, E, and C found in the pigment are natural antioxidants. These detox components are powerful and potent in boosting the body's internal detox platforms. Reducing toxins in the circulation is essential in controlling inflammation. Chlorophyll acts as an anti-inflammatory agent once it is degraded in the body. It can be used to treat chronic illnesses that are otherwise amenable to other forms of therapy. It is this ability to deal with inflammation that makes chlorophyll water very special, especially in cancer prevention.

When you take chlorophyll water as an alternative to soup from grains, meats, and nuts, you are protected from the toxins found in these types of foods. The other benefits of chlorophyll against cancer are as a result of the blockage of DNA damage from carcinogenic substances. Magnesium which is a chlorophyll-laden mineral is essential for cardiovascular, nervous, digestive, and musculoskeletal systems. The mineral helps improve conduction and blood supply together with oxygen delivery to the peripheral tissues. All the benefits of chlorophyll can be tapped from green drinks and green veggies. The advantage of taking chlorophyll water is that one is sure that the amounts of nutrients they are taking are on the higher side. Instead of making unhealthy juice recipes, it would be more healthful to throw in a few leaves of green plants to make chlorophyll water.

Juicing with Raw Fruits and Veggies

Juicing using fresh raw fruits and vegetables is very healthy and tasty. The mineral and vitamin content of fruit juices are extremely high and they can act as supplements in people leading a strict form of diet. You will boost your energy levels and get a variety of fruits in one glass. That's a great way to eat all your favorite fruits at once. Depending on your needs, you can make thick, creamy, or textured juices. To enrich your experience, have nutritious bases such as healthy nuts, soy, coconut, and dairies like milk or yoghurt. They are very effective in boosting the immune system and in helping the kidney by diuresis.

Smoothies are just as effective as juices from fruits and vegetable portions. People who prefer to juice veggies do so because they think that it is better to drink the vital sap from vegetables than to deal with the hard-to breakdown fibers. Fruit fibers are not as hard as those found in veggies and most people will prefer to take fruit smoothies. As long as you wash them properly, you are likely to get similar benefits from the juice and the smoothie.

However, it is true that fiber from smoothies adds more value in terms of aiding 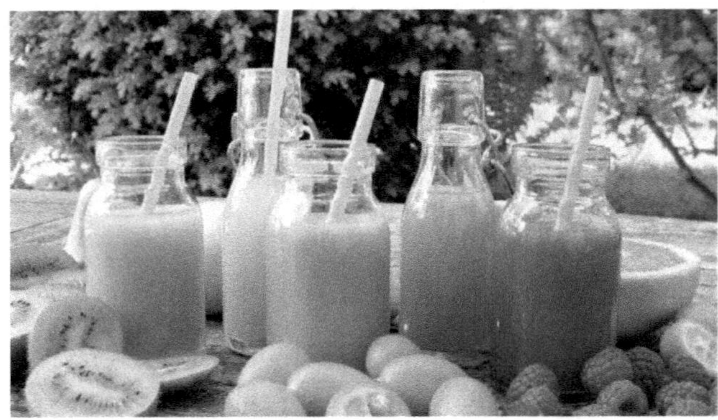 with digestion. Fruits with low water content like the banana, avocado, and papaya may not be the best for juicing and they need some extra water inside the blending machine. For juicing recipes, refer to our weight loss cookbook and get a variety of options.

Detox Fruits and Veggies

Many fruits and vegetables promise to offer nutrients and numerous health benefits. Some provide more than the nutrient factor and actually help in detoxifying the body. The name superfood is accorded to these vegetables and fruits since they offer more than what is in the face value. Below is a list of top 10 fruits and veggies that are potent detoxifiers:

1. **Avocado**- this fruit is a source of natural fats which are healthy for the body. It is a liver detoxifying fruit that works wonders in optimizing the function of the organ. Glutathione which helps in red cell metabolism is an important nutrient found in the avocado. It prevents the metabolism of unhealthy fats which are potential causes of toxins

2. **Beets**- for perfect liver cleansing, the beet should not miss in the diet. The red color of the food is made of anti-inflammatory

phytochemicals. It has both a detox and antifungal abilities which make it excellent in purging pathogens and their associated toxins.

3. **Cranberries**- Juicing using the cranberry is a great start in actively fighting the bacteria and boosting of the immune system. Rich in fiber and vitamins, it is an excellent way to stop hunger pangs when dieting. It also helps in weight loss since it has fewer calories.

4. **Grapes**- the grapefruit is known for its high fiber which cleanses the body from cholesterol and heavy metal poisons. It also acts on specific organs like the liver and the gut help in detoxifying the body.

5. **Kales**- add some finely chopped kale leaves into your salad and you won't regret the healthful choice. Kales have a reputation of detoxifying the body through the properties of phytochemicals and other antioxidants. It is also a great source of calcium and vitamin K and vitamin C.

6. **Cucumber**- the natural way of detoxifying the system using this fruit is made possible by its ability to flush away toxins in urine. It helps in dieresis and toxins are excreted with the water. It is also an anti-inflammatory food.

7. **Broccoli**- If you want to get a full dose of anti-oxidants, the broccoli is one way to go. Eating this green food helps one to mitigate the possibilities of having cancer. It is a rich source of protein and that is why it helps in weight loss.

8. **Cabbage**- cabbage can be eaten with anything cooked, or raw. You can throw in some of it into your smoothie to get the vitamins found in it. It is good for the liver and the gut since it helps in detoxifying the organ systems.

9. **Apples**- high water and fiber content of the apple fruit initiate and supports the process of losing weight. When you eat an apple, the normal flora in the gut is optimized and thus helps to keep the bad bacteria in check. As an antioxidant, be sure to deal a blow to diseases like diabetes type 2 and some types of heart diseases.

10. **Lemons**- You will rarely find any detox program lacking the lemon juice. It not only helps your gut to digest and absorb food contents but it also detoxifies and purges the system of toxins. Vitamin C in this fruit clears potentially dangerous chemicals from the body.

Detox Herbs and Spices

Herbs and spices add more than flavor to the taste of your food. People have used spices in food and beverages without the full knowledge of what they contain and their positive influence on healthy living. They boost the immunity and actively clear toxic metabolites from the body. Here is a list of top 10 herbs and spices that add value to your detox program:

1. **Ginger**- you can add ginger to flavor your smoothie but most importantly to provide detox. Ginger is anti-inflammatory and aids in digestion. Food transit in the gut increases favorably to flush off toxins.

2. **Cilantro**- for heavy metal elimination from the system, the cilantro works better than most of the herbs. It has an affinity for heavy metals such as lead and mercury and helps detox your body from such.

3. **Green tea**- you can take this herb in the form of tea or in a smoothie. Green tea has many benefits including diuresis to flush

toxins away and loss of weight since it has no calories. It is an antioxidant that helps the liver do a better work of toxin removal from the body.

4. **Cardamom**- going for a variety will land you the advantages of the cardamom spice. It is an antioxidant that binds free radicals preventing damage to the tissues. This makes it an anti-cancer spice that also helps in chronic diseases of the lungs, eyes, and teeth.

5. **Clove**- apart from its use in baking, clove is a bioactive spice with antioxidant characteristics. It helps in detoxifying and cleansing the body.

6. **Black Pepper**- the sour taste of pepper seems to be sour too to other species like bacteria. Moreover, pepper helps in congestion, toothaches, and constipation. It enhances sleep and optimizing the functionality of the individual.

7. **Cumin**- the cumin seeds have iron and other minerals. It is commonly used to reap its antiseptic, antioxidant, antifungal, laxative, antitumor, and carminative benefits. These properties can be achieved by adding it to food or applying it to the skin.

8. **Turmeric**- the important part of the turmeric is the curcumin which has antioxidant properties. It helps keep bacteria, fungi, and cancers at bay.

9. **Nutmeg**- the oils found in the nutmeg help people all over fight depression, digestive disturbances, oxidants, and other causes of toxic build up in the body.

10. **Chili**- to help in weight loss, add some chili t your food. It induces early satiety and you won't have to eat too much. It also helps detox

the body by binding free radicals thus preventing oxidative damage and aging of cells.

Most of the herbs, spices, vegetables, and fruits have multiple benefits and can be taken raw. This makes them suitable for all your juicing, smoothie, and tea needs. For healthy herbs and spices 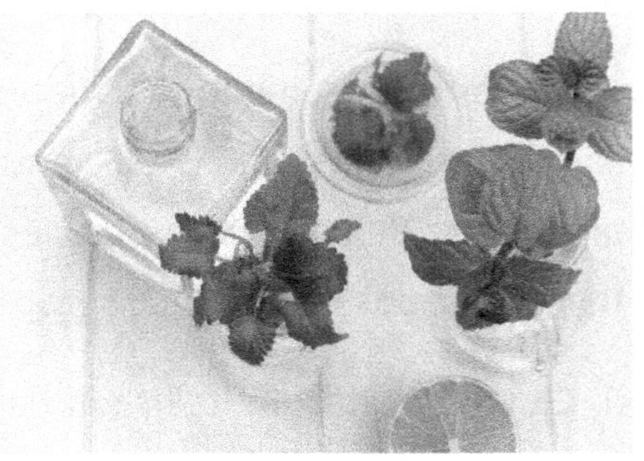 recipes, refer to our weight loss cookbook.

PHASE 2:
SHEDDING AND BURNING

Phase 2 is about shedding and burning. The guidelines indicated in this chapter should be strictly maintained throughout this phase. The length of the phase 2 will depend on the amount of weight you aim to lose and this can be calculated using the formula below. To get the length of stay in this phase, you will need to multiply the 1 week by the amount of kg you want to lose.

Phase 2 length (in weeks) = Amount of kg to lose

The ratio of nutrient consumption is;

Carbs : Proteins : Fats = 1 : 6 : 3

Proteins form the major part of the diet because you will need them during the intense workouts. As you shed calories, there is an increased need to build the muscle power and hence the need to take in more proteins. Fats are more than carbs in this phase to induce a ketogenic form of metabolism. This will train the body to effectively burn fats since it will be the main source of energy during this phase of the program.

Caloric intake = 800 calories for women
/1000 calories for men.

Once the body is in optimum mode, you can comfortably and efficiently burn calories and shed weight. It is the phase where most people find that they have to add some extra efforts into the weight loss program. The length of this phase can be short or long depending on the individual and the target weight. With all factors constant, you can achieve a weight loss of 1 kilo per week. This will mean that you can go for 12 weeks only if you want to cut 12 kg. To determine how much you need to lose to stay healthy, the individual needs to use the BMI or the WHR. Since the BMI is easy to use and the height will not change much, the weight loss target will be the amount of weight you need to shed to get to the BMI range of between 18.5 and 25 for men or 24.9 for women. If you are very obese, you should first target a BMI that will bring you to one level down in the BMI range. It is clear that the more the weight to cut, the longer they stay in phase 2. The great thing with this level is that it is a transition to a sure better life. You could use the following to get the weight of your dreams;

- Intermittent Fasting
- Low carb intake
- Low fat intake
- High protein diet
- Enough fiber consumption
- Probiotics
- Supplementation

All the listed interventions have a positive impact on weight loss. A combination of some of them leads to a sustainable burning of calories. You will need all the motivation to stay in this phase. Most times the weight cut is favorable and encourages the individual to keep going. You will have to stick to the program for at least a few weeks to see a significant change in the scale.

Intermittent Fasting

The 16/8 Intermittent Fasting

	Sunday	Monday	Tuesday	Wednesday	Thursday	Friday	Saturday	Sunday
12 pm (Mid-day)	Not fasting	Not fasting	Eat	Not fasting	Eat	Not fasting	Eat	Not fasting
4 pm	Not fasting	Not fasting	Eat	Not fasting	Eat	Not fasting	Eat	Not fasting
8 pm	Not fasting	Not fasting	Fast	Not fasting	Fast	Not fasting	Fast	Not fasting
12 am	Sleep	Sleep	Fast (Sleep)	Sleep	Fast (sleep)	Sleep	Fast (sleep)	Sleep
4 am	Sleep	Sleep	Fast (Sleep)	Sleep	Fast (sleep)	Sleep	Fast (sleep)	Sleep
8 am	Not fasting	Not fasting	Fast (awake)	Not fasting	Fast (awake)	Not fasting	Fast (awake)	Not fasting

Mondays are busy days for most people since they have to go to work and perform a couple of activities. You may also feel lazy after a long weekend and fasting may become a problem. It is better to schedule Tuesday, Thursday, and Saturday as fasting days.

Intermittent fasting plans do no more than changing your eating pattern. The 16/8 intermittent fasting program for instance simply changes and restricts your eating time to a period of 8 hours. The rest of your 24- hour day is fasting time. It doesn't need much of a struggle because we naturally fast for most of the night when we are asleep. You will shed weight through burning excess fat when the body is forced to stay without food for some time. Much of your muscle tissue is spared or even increased during the schedule. A fast lasting for less than 8-12 hours is not effective in losing weight as much. You need to get out of the post-absorptive state and enter the fasting state of the body's metabolism. Insulin levels go low when the body is fasting and the other hormones come into play to ensure that you utilize the stored calories.

When you decide to go induce a fasting mode, your day is made simpler since the hustle of preparing meals is reduced. You may just take water and hit the road as you wait for the feeding window. There are many models of fasting using the 16/8 plan and all you have to do is choose the days that you wish to skip some of your meals in the day. Daily intermittent fasting is possible although not very necessary because it is unhealthy. It adds stress which causes you to overeat to feel better. Stress hormones build up and insulin secretion is increased. The blood glucose levels fall as sugars are stored up and you crave for more food and you end up getting fat. You can choose to fast in 3 days and eat regularly during the rest of the days in a week.

Convenience is key in formulating a lasting fasting plan. Which meals can you eat alone and which ones need everyone at the family table? The meals that can be altered are those that do not interfere with the program of the rest of the family members. You can choose to eat during an 8-hour period between noon and dusk to accommodate the need to have lunch and dinner as a family. This will leave you with a 16-hour fasting period that spans through the night when you are asleep and part of your morning. Refer to the sample IF plan given above and if the days mentioned seem impossible or inconvenient, then arrange it with your own easy days.

Tips

- *Choose the days in which you feel most comfortable*
- *Don't sleep around for the entire 16 hours of fasting*
- *Be active and do your duties as you would when you have eaten*
- *Withhold food but not healthy drinks during the fast so that you stay hydrated*
- *Water is the preferred type of fluid*
- *You can take other drinks such as teas and juices with a minimal calorie count*
- *Before breaking the fast, burn more calories by doing a low intensive workout*
- *Break the fast first with a juice or a smoothie and then eat harder food later*
- *The eating period should take care of your cravings, so that you get a smooth fasting period*
- *If hunger is intolerable, break the fast, solve the problem, and then schedule for another fast*

Low Carb Foods

For most people, carbs form a major almost irreplaceable part of their diets. High carb content is responsible for much of the weight gain because the body doesn't need as much as we eat. To shed weight, the individual needs to look for ways to reduce the total carb intake in the diet. This may involve using tools such as the glycemic index.

What is the Glycemic Index?

In simple terms, the glycemic index is the value of your carb foods. Not all foods have an equal amount of calories or ability to be digested and absorbed into the bloodstream. Using this fact, the glycemic index helps in determining the individual ranking of a carbohydrate-based on how fast or slow it leads to a change in the blood sugars. Foods such as apples and bananas have lower glycemic indices compared to potatoes and white rice. The carb-containing foodstuffs with a low glycemic index are better choices of low-calorie foods. They are slowly digested and metabolized and hence they don't lead to an increased glucose burden in the body. Low indexed foods have a glycemic index of less than 55, while moderately indexed foods have between 56 and 69. Potatoes and other foods with high-carb content have their glycemic indices at more than 70.

Food	Calorie count per 100g
Bread whole meal	220
Maraconi	95
Noodles (boiled)	70
pasta (boiled)	110
white rice (boiled)	140
porridge oats (with water)	55
spaghetti (boiled)	101

What you should eat

You can eat the carbohydrates with low glycemic index since they don't lead to much weight problems. Whole grains, legumes, fruits, and gluten-free foods have low glycemic indices and release their glucose slowly and steadily. Eating such types of foods helps in maintaining the energy levels over a longer time without the risk of storing excess calories. If you must sweeten your food or drinks, opt for honey or artificial sweeteners which have a low glycemic index.

Food	Calorie count per 100g
Potatoes	140
Chapattis	300
Cream crackers	440
Biscuit digestives	480

What you shouldn't eat

There are no-go-zones when it comes to taking low carb foods. It is better to avoid foods with high glycemic indices than to eat them in smaller proportions. Refined sugars, corn syrup, mashed or boiled potatoes, sweets, cakes, pastries are all sources of a high-calorie level. These types of carbohydrates are not the best for weight loss. They will keep you on a plateau and you will have to struggle to hit the 1 kg per week target.

Low Fat Food

Low-fat foods are good for weight loss and many manufacturers are making such foods. Unfortunately, fat is very essential in offering food its great taste and the manufacturers move to salvage the situation by adding more sugar and salt to the food products. This makes the low-fat foods unhealthier and a bad option for the individual who needs to shed calories.

Food	Calorie count per 100g
Low fat spread	400
Avocado	150 (per piece)
Lobster	100
Chia seeds	486
Tuna	180

What you should eat

Avocado, seafood, fish, coconut oil, and olive oil are good sources of fat. The type of fat contains omega 3 which has numerous health benefits such as boosting the immunity and the energy levels. Avocado and fish are easily affordable fatty food sources that should be regular in your weight loss diet. Extra virgin oil, extra virgin coconut oil, and plates of seafood may be difficult to get in the diet as frequently as one would have wished. Maximize on the available sources and seize the opportunities of the rare sources when they present. Low-fat milk with no added flavors or refined sugars can be used as an alternative to full cream milk.

Food	Calorie count per 100g
Pork	290
Mutton (thigh)	224
Butter	750
Ghee (clarified butter)	876
Margarine	750
Pure fat	900

What you shouldn't eat

Foods that are guaranteed to ruin your weight loss include pork, mutton, trans fat, butter, cream, ghee, corn oil, and palm oil. They are loaded with unhealthy fats and no matter how much the manufacturer may want to reduce the fat content, it still remains dangerously high. Avoid these sources of fats and get a desirable progress in shedding weight. There are many more great sources of natural and healthy fat which one can choose from.

Consuming Protein Rich Foods

Food	Calorie count per 100g
Beef	
Chicken	280
Liver	200
Salmon	300
Fish cake	180
Fish fingers	200
Sardines	220
tinned	220
Egg hard	155
boiled	80
Beans baked	

Meat

Proteins are body-building foods and meats have high levels of this vital nutrient. Grass-fed beef and organic chicken provide very high percentages of an individual's daily recommendation. When all the fat layers and skin are removed from the meat, you remain with an even higher protein level source. Workouts can drain the muscle power and health. Recovery without the intake of adequate proteins in severely intense workouts may prove difficult since the muscle mass is reduced under such environments. In fact, the more you workout, the more you should add double portions of proteins in the diet. This is the only way to survive the hours of training at the gym to burn fat. Increasing the muscle power through taking good amounts of proteins helps you become more suitable at burning calories. The other direct advantage derived from a high protein diet is that the intake of alternative foods such as carbs and fats reduce as does the total calorie input into the system.

Fish

Wild caught fish like the salmon provide high amounts of proteins and omega fats which are much needed in healthy weight loss. You don't get the problems of undernutrition when you have salmon in the diet. It helps in the growth and development of almost all the organ systems with a particular emphasis on the brain, bones, heart, skin, and eyes.

Egg whites without the yolk *(52 calories per 100 grams)*

Remove the yolk of the egg which is full of cholesterol and you remain with a full profile of amino acids in your diet. Eggs also have vitamin B6 that helps in protein metabolism. The eggs from a free-range hen are better in protein value and lower in fat calorie.

Food	Calorie count per 100g
Lentils	100
Kidney beans	127

Lentils and Kidney Beans

Vegetarians know the value of lentils and kidney beans than most other people. Beans are great protein sources with high fiber content. The fiber makes you feel full over longer periods and your eating frequency is reduced to foster weight loss. The legumes are also known for their extremely low glycemic index in the food list. Proteins in lentils are high enough to sustain the strict vegetarian needs.

Consume Enough Fiber

Leafy fruits, oats, and vegetables provide a lot of fiber in the diet. Fiber works to relieve constipation which can get you ill and unable to pass stool. Dietary fiber is also known as roughage and is made up of the indigestible food parts which are ingested to get many health benefits. The fiber is not absorbed and remains throughout the bowels until it is excreted. Fiber from the diet could either be soluble or insoluble with the solvent being water.

Both types of fiber are important in their own different and unique ways. Taking soluble fiber helps in lowering the cholesterol levels.

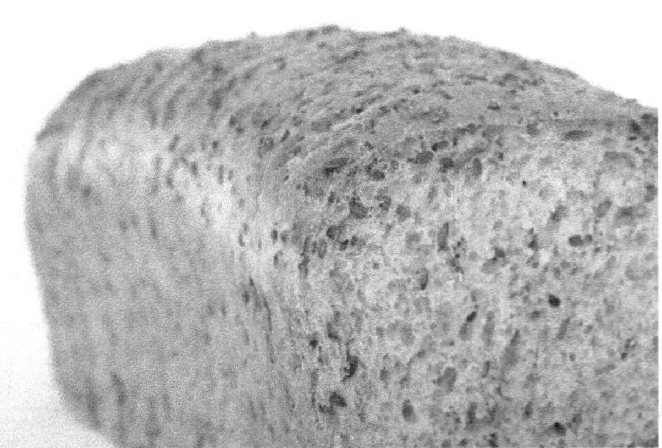

It dissolves in water and becomes like a paste that passes down the gut. Insoluble fiber is good for bulk formation helping with the transit of other food contents along the alimentary canal. If you want this type of fiber to relieve chronic constipation, eat foods such as whole wheat flour, bran, beans, whole veggies, fruits, and nuts. You need a normal bowel movement to allow you to maneuver the gym moves as you do your workouts. Irregular bowel habits can ruin your peace, schedule, and sleep hygiene.

Probiotics

Probiotics are living micro-organisms such as bacteria and yeasts that are found in foods such as yoghurt (lactobacillus). Fermented foods and supplements with live commensals and symbiotic organisms are

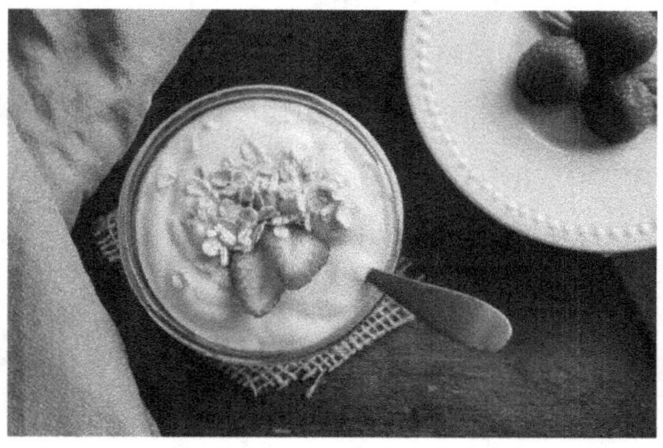

some of the options for Probiotics. The good bacteria keep the bad bacteria from multiplying in the body. This improves the gut health and leads to loss of weight. The organisms may inhibit fat absorption and reduce the calories from such sources which end up being excreted and not absorbed. Your body will only absorb a small amount of the fats which is all you need. The Probiotics could help in the release of hormones that make you feel full or those that antagonize the signal to store fat.

Supplementation

Vitamins and Antioxidants are needed to boost the metabolism which favors weight loss. Antioxidants block the pathways of toxic reactants in the body by actually oxidizing them. Oxygen in certain levels as in free radicals can be damaging and it is the job of vitamins and antioxidants to protect the body. Supplementing the dietary intake of vitamins and micronutrients is required in weight loss. It helps boost the ability of the body to fight toxins. This is why you need herbs and spices such as turmeric and green tea.

The Vitamin B complex is necessary for your body to have a fully optimized metabolism. It helps the individual to burn calories from by enhancing the metabolism of fats, carbs, and proteins. Your body will be in a better position to use stored calories. Vitamin D is lower in obese people, an indicator that it is essential for weight loss. Supplementing vitamin D if you can't get enough from the food or sun helps burn abdominal fat. Vitamin C aids in the absorption of food to support the increased metabolic demands.

PHASE 3: MAINTAINING THE HEALTHY WEIGHT

The specific guidelines for phase 3 of maintaining the healthy weight span over your lifetime. You need to stick to the recommendations so that you consolidate the gains of the program and stay healthy all through your life.

Phase 2 length = Lifetime

Limit the Calorie Intake

Many people having weight problems while eating healthy foods do not have a control over the portion size. The total caloric intake matters a lot in weight loss and maintenance of a healthy weight. You begin the calorie limit in this phase and maintain it for your lifetime. The change in the caloric intake from the previous phase is to maintain the lost weight in a healthy way.

Maximum calorie intake = 1200 calories for women /1500 calories for men.

The required daily caloric intake is about 1000-1200 calories in women. Men could eat more with no potential weight problems but they should never eat beyond 1200-1500 calories per day. Men have more muscle and can burn more calories than women. Special states such as pregnancy or athletic professions may require one to take more calories.

The recommended ratio of macronutrients aligns with the in the Harvard healthy eating plate i=during this phase and it is;

$$\textbf{Carbs : Proteins : Fats = 2 : 4 : 1}$$

Every meal should get close to the ratio of a balanced nutrition and the healthy eating plate tries to achieve it.

Do Not Skip Breakfast

This phase is the maintenance phase. You will consume 3 meals and 2 snacks in the recommended portion sizes. The breakfast is the meal that must never be skipped when you want to maintain your body weight. It gives you get a replenishment of sugars which get used up at night which is much needed by the body and the brain. A good breakfast should have enough energy to push you through the day. This will boost your metabolism and prevent hunger and fatigue before it is time for lunch. Skipping breakfast leads to an increase in stress hormone cortisol. This will make you get a cranky feeling and a slowed metabolism which will lead to poor weight control.

Unlike in phase 2, you will not be following an intermittent fasting plan in this phase of program, because you aim at maintaining rather than losing the weight. Therefore, it is necessary to take your meals and fill them with all healthy food.

8-Hours of Regular Sleep

Sleeping for 8 hours every day is needed to control stress. You will get problems if you either sleep too much or too little. Sleep debt must be paid through dozing in the day at work of postponing the gym time to take an afternoon nap. To avoid problems that can impair your metabolism or ability to work out, have a good night's sleep of about 8 hours daily. Supplements in maintenance phase need not be given as regularly as in the previous phases. The metabolism is already boosted and working optimally. Doing two-week supplementation every month is enough to keep you going.

Harvard Healthy Eating Plate

After all the hustle and struggles to lose weight, there is a greater need to maintain it healthy. It is the phase that makes all the difference sometimes. Most likely, it will involve a complete turnaround of the individual's life, lifestyle choices, and habits. The phase involves making the healthy habits part of your life. To maintain a healthy weight, you may need to use the Harvard healthy eating plate.

The healthy eating plate design is an improvement to the USDA's MyPlate. It is a simple and detailed format to follow in making the right eating choices. The plate is divided into four unequal quadrants with the healthier foods taking up a bigger portion than the rest. Using the guide helps you make choices on breakfast, lunch, dinner, and snacks. You should eat healthy fruits as much as possible. They have low calories and high fiber content which is good for gut functioning and provision of enough energy. Plenty of fruits means that a day should not go without you taking some fruits during meals.

Ideally, they should be part of every meal although it may be difficult to achieve this scenario.

Veggies and greens in a variety make the greatest percent of the healthy eating plate. You need to be creative and ensure that they come in all the variety that nature provides. Potatoes and potato foods like French fries are vegetables but they do not count in the portion. Pick healthy vegetables that offer enough nutrition to avoid deficiency syndromes. The greens can be taken raw in salads or cooked. When preparing the veggies, you should use healthy oils otherwise you will counteract the health benefits conferred by these foods. Olive oil and canola oils are the recommended oils. Butter can be used but trans fats should never be used to prepare your foods.

Whole grains in all their vast varieties such as whole wheat bread, grain pasta, and brown rice are good for maintaining a healthy weight. Whole grains also have fiber and you won't have constipation. They are advantageous over the processed grains with hulls removed. Healthy proteins include anything that is free from high-fat content. Fish, poultry, beans, nuts are the great protein sources that should frequent your diet. Red meat and cheese may be taken in moderation but bacon, and other processed meat products should not be consumed in the healthy Harvard plate.

Drink lots of fluids with little or no added sugar. Water, tea, and coffee are good for hydrating the body and helping with digestion. Sugary drinks such as carbonated drinks won't help you maintain a good weight. Drink milk and dairy products once in a while with no more than 1 or 2 servings per day. Remember to stay active too so that the excess calories don't build up in the body and cause you to regain weight.

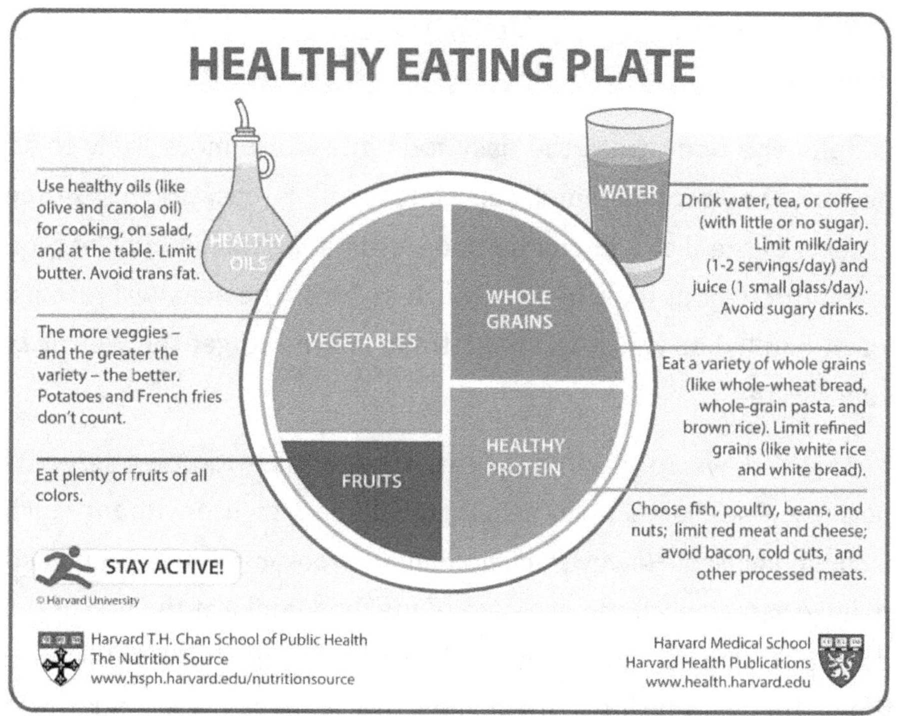

Never Return Back to Your Old Self

Cravings may come and be so strong as to cause you to desire the previous unhealthy life. You should never go back to the unhealthy lifestyle after making progressive weight loss. Regaining weight will discourage any further motives to stay healthy. It will also make you unfit to handle the exercises that effectively burnt your excess calories.

Food Diary (Tracking)

Keeping a diary of every food item you eat can make all the difference in weight loss. Trying to maintain a certain weight without tabling the food measures is difficult. It is only through the diary that an individual can get to the core of the weight problem. Knowing the right food to eat in weight dieting is the initial step that requires a follow-up on the quantity and even quality of these foods.

People who don't track the daily food intake are more likely to go beyond the recommended daily intakes. It is easy to miss some aspects of the diet and end up underestimating the amount of food taken throughout the day by as much as 50 %. The diary will reveal a lot of bad habits which will need to be altered to get the weight of your desire.

It doesn't have to be a complicated diary since it won't serve its purpose. The diary should be simple and easy to use without much inconveniencing. However, it shouldn't be too simple since you need to have a near- accurate estimate of the food intake at the end of the day. You will need to record not only the serving size but also the meal times. This will help localize problems such as excess food intake after dinner or during the breakfast. Sometimes the problem is with eating less during certain times of the day leading to more hunger and impulse to eat unhealthy snacks.

The aim of tracking your food intake is to be accountable. Using the diary, you can get the sources of plateaus in the dieting plan and improve on them. The diary should be recorded frequently if possible and not at the end of the day since you might forget a snack or a drink taken in between meals. To lose and maintain weight, you will have to record the meal habits of at least 3 days every week.

After keeping a record of your feeding diary, you will realize that you need to make some changes in the food types and quantities. A healthy weight pyramid is useful in accomplishing this task. It ensures that your choice of foods is healthy in that you eat less from the top of the pyramid and more from the bottom. Sweet foods such as candy, cakes, cookies, and pies should be least recorded while vegetables and fruits should be most recorded in the diary.

The servings in the food diary should be recorded to estimate the number of nutrients which you eat on a daily basis. 5 or more servings for vegetables and fruits, 4 for carbohydrates, 4 for proteins or dairy, and 3 for fats is ideal for the individual who does a little exercise. The diary should be tailored to meet the needs of the dieter. For instance, having a slot for exercises will make the tool more valuable.

Get the daily food tracking sheet printed to record your progress;

Daily Food Tracking Sheet		
	Servings/calories	Comments
Breakfast		
Vegetables		
Fruits		
Grains		
Lean proteins		
Other proteins		
Healthy fats		
Water/fluid		
Lunch		
Vegetables		
Fruits		
Grains		
Lean proteins		
Other proteins		
Healthy fats		
Water/fluid		
Dinner		
Vegetables		
Fruits		
Grains		
Lean proteins		
Other proteins		
Healthy fats		
Water/fluid		
Snacks		
Vegetables		
Fruits		
Grains		
Lean proteins		
Other proteins		
Healthy fats		
Water/fluid		

PART 3

THE WORKOUT GUIDE

BURNING FAT WITH WORKOUT

Excess body fat has been documented to be associated with the risk of development of a lot of health problems such as diabetes, depression, cardiac diseases and some forms of cancer. As a result, many people seek means to shed this fat. When combined properly with a scale back on unhealthy food, exercise is the most important step towards burning fat.

The body normally stores up energy in the form of fat when one consumes food and uses less energy than that gotten from the food for the daily metabolism. If one consistently consumes more calories than one utilises over a long period of time, the fat stores continue to build up. During exercise, the body needs fuel in the form a compound known as ATP; this is easily derived from the sugar stores in the body. With fairly rigorous exercise, the sugar stores in the muscles are rapidly depleted and the body then turns to its fat reserves which are converted to sugar that can then be used to generate the fuel required for the exercise. The exercise has to be of a sufficiently rigorous nature in order to ensure that the body has to resort to its fat stored to generate fuel.

Measuring BMI and hip-waist ratio

An objective way of assessing the amount of fat in the body is the system known as the Body Mass Index (BMI). The BMI is a measure of the amount of tissue mass (muscle, fat and bone) in adult males and women which then acts as an indicator of the amount of fat in a person's body. As the BMI of an individual increases, so does the total body fat of such an individual. Obtaining the 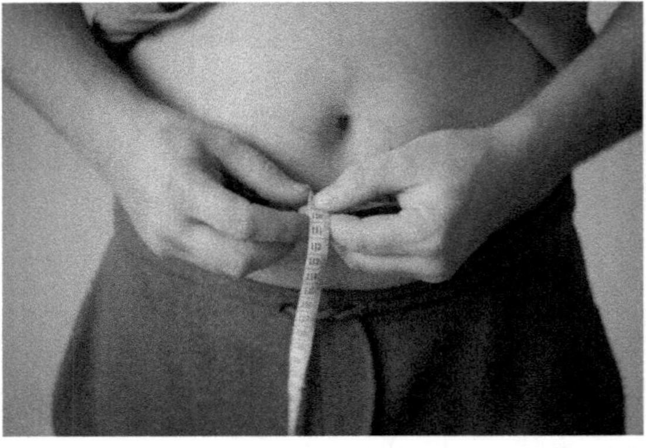 BMI requires an accurate assessment of an individual's weight and height which are then computed to get this index.

To obtain an accurate assessment of body weight, the first step is to purchase a weighing scale of which there are the analogue and digital forms. The digital weighing scales are generally more accurate than the analogue ones as a result of the easy occurrence of errors of parallax while reading analogue scales and the precision to which digital scales can read weight. Analogue forms are almost as good. The reading obtained on a scale can vary based on how much clothing one has on, how much food or water has been ingested as well as the time of day. To ensure accurate and consistent results, weigh yourself in your bathroom when there are no clothes on, the weighing should also be done at the same time every day; perhaps on waking up before having any food or drink. The scale should be placed on a flat surface to ensure an accurate reading. Calibrating the scale is also important and a scale will come with a manual which explains how this can be done.

The other component of the BMI is the height and this also has to be measured accurately. The stadiometer is the gold standard for measuring height. Just as good is the use of the wall height in which you stand up straight against the walls, the feet together and the back of the head, calves and back of the feet in contact with the wall. An observer then helps to note the highest point of the head which is then taken as the height.

$$BMI= [Weight(kg) \div height\ (m^2)]$$

BMI	Interpretation
Less than 18.5	Underweight
18.5 – 24.9	Normal
25 – 29.9	Overweight
30 - 35	Obesity class 1
35 - 40	Obesity class 2
More than 40	Obesity class 3

A value less than 18.5 is underweight, between 18.5 and 24.9 is normal, between 25 and 29.9 is overweight while values between 30 and 35 are classified as Class 1 Obesity, those between 35 and 40 as Class 2 Obesity while BMI values greater than 40 regarded as Class 3 obesity.

WHR Norms				
Gender	Healthy	Good	Average	Unhealthy
Female	<0.8	0.75-0.79	0.8-0.89	>0.9
Male	<0.9	0.85-0.89	0.9-0.99	>1

The hip-waist ratio is another means of evaluating body fat and obesity. The girth of the waist is taken as that obtained just above the belly button while the hip's girth is measured at the most prominent point of the buttocks with the individual standing straight and relaxed. Measurement should be done with a non-expansible tape measure and repeat measurements should use the same landmark. Hip-waist ratios of less than 0.8 and 0.9 are considered normal in females and males respectively while values greater than this are regarded as being overweight.

With the Body Mass Index or Hip-waist ratio determined, an assessment of just about how much fat an individual has stored up can be made and this can be used to set a goal on how to establish a workout routine that works.

S	Specific
M	Measurable
A	Attainable
R	Realistic
T	Time bound

What is the goal?

As with any other life project, it is crucial to have a set of goals to be achieved within a timeframe. It is not just enough to aim to burn fat with workout, it is essential to have particular goals as to how much weight you want to lose in a given time, how much work you will put in everyday to attain the goal and possible rewards when the goal is attained. A well-established mnemonic for setting objectives is the SMART criterion which is shown in the table below:

Deciding to become healthier is a broad goal while deciding to go about it by working out is already a specific goal. It can be made even more specific by deciding what workout routines will be embarked on (aerobics, anaerobics) as well as how long to invest daily. Having established the need to work out and the work out plan, the progress of the process has to be measured and tracked- in this instance, you can keep track of how long you have exercised in a day with a notebook or fitness tracker as well as how your weight has changed over a period of time. The goals should be made attainable and realistic- there is no point attempting a 20 kilometre run on your first try, instead, aim at starting with easier targets that can then be gradually increased. Having realistic goals might mean that results will take a while to be apparent, so it is essential to be able to keep at exercising even when the results are not apparent. Create a time frame in which you want to burn a certain amount of fat and then create how to do it. This can be easily documented in a journal to ensure that adequate attention is paid to detail.

Other important considerations in setting workout goals are incorporating exercises which you find exciting into your routine, this increases the likelihood of completing them. Also, check with a physician if you have chronic health issues to ensure that the workout routine is personalised.

Choose the Right Time for You

Consistency is an important tool to burn fat via workout. A crucial step is exercising daily and choosing the duration of exercise to be embarked on as well as at what time of the day. It has been shown that it takes between 15 and 20 minutes for the body to use up its normal sugar reserves after which it starts 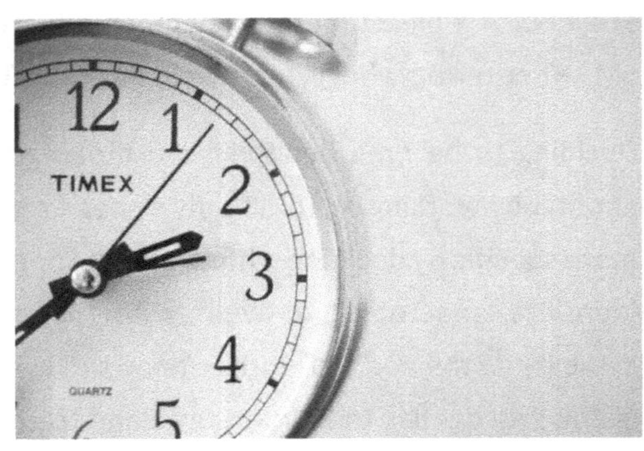 converting fat to sugar. To take advantage of this fact, exercise can be tailored to be between 30 minutes and 1 hour every day. The next step is choosing whether to exercise in the morning or during the rest of the day, this time should be fixed in order to build a routine. The time most generally advocated is an early morning workout for numerous reasons. First, it helps to minimise potential clashes of the exercise routine with other life activities that might pop up unexpected during the day. Also, the body is most likely in a fasted state when one has just woken up meaning that there are lower sugar reserves to call on and the fat begins to burn much faster. The fatigue that comes with the stress of daily life is also eliminated. In addition, blood levels of cortisol, a fat burning stress hormone are at very high levels in the morning and this further helps to burn fat. However, exercising early in the morning necessitates a high protein diet to avoid loss of muscle mass.

In addition to these benefits, exercise has been shown to improve the levels of circulating serotonin in the blood stream. Serotonin is a chemical which transmits messages within the brain and has effects on mood, appetite and alertness. Higher levels have the added advantage of reducing the risk of depression and can be achieved by choosing a morning routine which helps to keep serotonin levels up all day long.

In the event that you have little time to spend on working out, avoid the temptation of striking out your workout session from your schedule. Instead, you can try a number of tricks both to create more time and to utilise the available time effectively. First, try waking up fifteen to twenty minutes earlier than usual to get that bit of more time, you can try running or cycling to work instead of taking the commute or try lunchtime exercises at work. You can also work on increasing the intensity of your normal routine by running faster over a shorter period of time.

In your workout routine, start with moves that you dislike and work towards those you might be anticipating, this helps to motivate you and shortens the time spent. Finally, try high intensity-interval trainings such as the Tabata training- it consists of eight rounds of ultra-high-intensity exercises in a specific 20-seconds-on, 10-seconds-off interval spread over four minutes. It has been shown to be an effective means of working out within a short time interval.

COMMON MISTAKES OF WEIGHT LOSS WORKOUTS

Many people start weight loss workout plans, but only a few successfully complete them. This is due to numerous mistakes they do during their weight loss workout programs. Starting from the errors of how they set a goal to the amount and intensity of workouts they carry out can determine how successful you can be. Let us now have a look at a few common mistakes people do during their workout programs.

☐ **Beginning gym workouts without a solid plan:**

It is very important to figure out what and how you want to exert yourself at the gym. You will not be achieving your weight loss goals by simply hitting the gym. There should be a specific plan which indicates which type of exercises you will do and the number of repetitions should be pre-planned. This will help you to focus on the plan and to achieve successful;results.

☐ **Repeating same exercises every day.**

It is very important to train all your body rather than one part of your body to achieve weight loss. If you are planning to repeat the same exercises, you are very far from achieving weight loss goal that you have in your mind. Further, repeating same exercises every day, you will feel bored and eventually lose the motivation to lose weight.

Your main goal is not only to achieve a targeted weight, but also to obtain a good shape. In order to do this, it is important that you include different exercises in different cycles so that you will not spare any hidden fat deposits.

☐ **Not giving sufficient rest.**

Your body needs rest to repair the sore muscles following workout. If you do not give yourself enough time to rest, your muscles can become sore and lead to injury. This in turn increases the time taken to reach your weight loss goal. And also, insufficient rest also increases the body's stress and thus, it can actually lead to weight gain.

☐ **Performing cardio as the only workout.**

Cardio exercises are definitely helpful to build your stamina and burn calories. But, strength training exercises are those that help in building muscles and shaping up the body. Actually, strength training and cardio alone cannot give you that zero size or shaped body. For that it is necessary to enrol in stretching and also body balancing workouts. A complex combination of these exercises can only reach you to the goal of achieving a well shaped body.

☐ **Forgetting pre and post workout meals**

Most people forget about pre and post workout meals. They prefer to go on an empty stomach to start their workout. Pre and post workout meals are high essential to enable the body to perform workout as well as to repair. This is scientifically proven. Anyhow, this doesn't mean that you should have a heavy meal before your workouts. But, the best way to begin a workout is by drinking a little water and having a high protein, very low calorie snack. The same should be repeated after your workouts. Rest for about 10 minutes after your workouts and let your heart rate reduces before you eat or drink anything. Post workout fluid intake should be more as you have sweated a lot.

☐ **Performing improper technique**

If you are not using proper technique when exercising, you won't be able to get the maximum benefit out of it. In addition, improper techniques also lead to injury instead of weight loss. Therefore, learn the techniques first, warm up and then enrol in your workouts.

PHASE 1:
DETOXIFYING & BOOSTING

The process of burning fat via exercise can be looked at in three phases, the first of which is discussed in this chapter- this is the boosting phase. The other phases- the burning and shedding and maintenance phases are discusses in subsequent chapters.

The How To

In the boosting phase, the general aim is to increase fitness and build strength and resistance which will allow participation in long workouts as the exercises become more tedious. This phase can be achieved by working and jogging, which are aerobic exercises, more commonly referred to as cardio. Aerobic exercises are exercises in which oxygen is adequate to meet the energy demands of such exercises. Anaerobic exercise on the other hand increases the rate at which sugar is broken down, this leads to the build-up of lactate in muscles which causes pain in the muscles and can eventually lead to nausea and vomiting. For this to be avoided, the exercises are usually of a low to medium intensity and thus do not have high energy demands. Other cardio exercises include rowing, running on a treadmill and using a stationary bicycle. Outdoor walking and jogging however are perhaps the easiest to stick to and can be easier to stick to.

These cardio exercises have a range of benefits of which an increase in metabolic rate is the most pertinent for the person trying to burn fat. Jogging and running raise the amount of 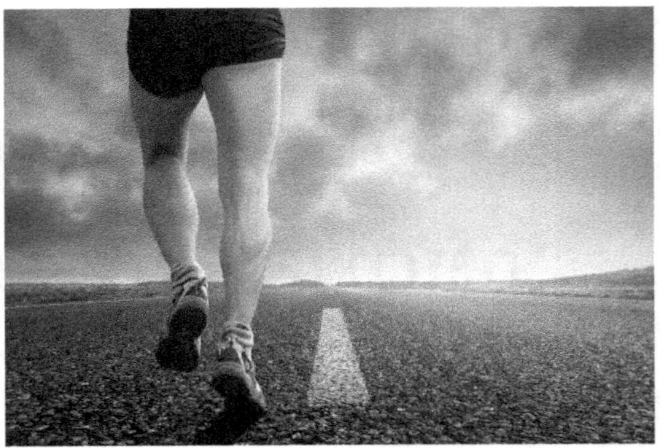 energy needed to sustain the body cells and the body, in a bit to meet up with the increased metabolic rate resorts to breakdown of fats to supply the energy needed. A person weighing 50kg will burn about 180 calories when jogging for 30 minutes which represents a significantly increased metabolic rate. Other benefits include improving the ability of cells to utilise fat for energy, strengthening the body's muscles of respiration which in the long run allows one to exercise for longer periods as well as causing increased blood levels from increased erythropoietin levels.

The duration of walking and jogging is another very important consideration. It is generally advisable to run at a moderate pace for periods of 25 to 30 minutes daily. With time, respiratory capacity to carry out aerobic exercise is built and endurance is obtained. Thus, the jogging speed can be gradually increased every day at a low rate to allow easy acclimatisation and avoid the risk of overuse injury. As running only increases the metabolic rate for short periods of time, it is advisable to keep at it daily to ensure the maximal effect.

The table below shows the average number of calories burnt per 30 minutes for the highlighted Vary your walking workout to keep it interesting and you will also burn more calories.

Excersice	Calories Burnt per 30 minutes
Walking	90 – 100
Brisk walking	120 – 140
Jogging	250 – 290
Running	300 - 350

As the aim of these exercises is to allow the body to burn calories, it is advisable to incorporate a couple of inclines into your walking route by walking along hilly terrains. If you exercise on a treadmill, set it at a slope for about half of the workout time. Walking more extreme inclines burns twice the amount of calories than walking on a flat route as the effect of the incline is as though one were on a hike.

Picking the right shoes with which to jog is perhaps just as important as making the decision to jog as it helps reduce the risk of injuries and provides comfort and the right amount of spring while running. First, consider the surface on which you will run to determine how much traction and cushion is needed on the shoes. Lighter shoes will work well with road running while trail or mountain running requires shoes with more cushion and traction to accommodate the uneven surfaces that will be encountered.

The other factor which determines the type of shoe to purchase is the type of foot you possess. Three kinds of feet are broadly recognised- neutral feet, overpronation and underpronation. Individuals with neutral feet have feet which touch the ground around the middle of the foot and should go for shoes made for neutral runners which have no accommodations to counteract pronation. An overweight neutral runner might however consider a shoe with a modest degree of support and cushion. Overpronators have feet that roll inward and should go for shoes designed to maintain stability and improve motion control. Underpronators have feet which roll outwards and should go for shock absorbing and cushioned shoes. It is advisable to pick up a running shoe from the local store instead of purchasing online as it allows you to pick the right size and sales representatives can provide help on the right shoe for you. Consider a shoe that is a half size larger to accommodate for slight swellings in the foot that may occur with running.

Running in places with fresh air helps provide a serene environment to relax and ensures adequate oxygen intake to keep exercise aerobic. Trail running might entail various up and down movements which even helps burn fat faster

PHASE 2:
BURNING AND SHEDDING

The next phase after boosting strength and endurance is the actual burning and shedding of weight. It is a phase of extreme hard work for which a dedication to the set goal is required. Exercise that can help to burn and shed the fat entails:

Intense Aerobic/Cardio workouts

Intensity is essential to the process of burning fat and more calories are burned as the intensity of exercise increases. Cardio exercises are crucial to the process of burning fat as they increase the metabolism rate to a greater amount over short periods of time while also increasing the calorie deficit. They also serve to keep the heart healthy to ensure that regular exercise is easy. The specific goals of cardio exercise are:

- ☐ To burn calories
- ☐ To increase overall stamina
- ☐ To improve heart and lung function (circulation)
- ☐ To manage other health risks such as hypertension and diabetes.

A variety of exercise options exist that serve as aerobic workouts including:

Running: The benefits of running have been described earlier and with a higher intensity of running, even more fat is burned.

Elliptical: This simulates walking and running while

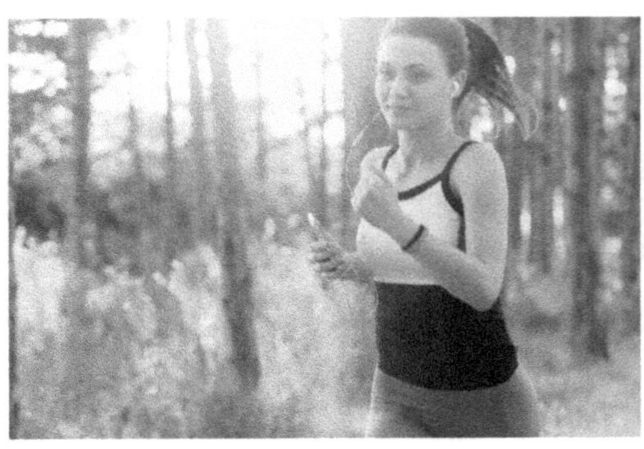

reducing the risk of injuries by avoiding stress on the joints. Increasing the incline of the machine can also help simulate the process of stair climbing and help burn more fats. One set of about 20 minutes three times a week is sufficient to burn a lot of fat. It is also essential to ensure that the arms are not doing most of the work by avoiding holding on to the rails too tightly. Ellipticals can burn as much as 600 calories in an hour.

Cycling: This utilises pretty much the same set of muscles involved in running while being less demanding and more fun. Cycling daily for about 20-30 minutes can serve as an intense form of cardio burning as much as 400 calories in 20 minutes.

Skipping: Skipping is an easy exercise which also comes with the benefits of lesser cost. It helps to burn a lot of calories and also has the added advantage of improving balance and coordination.

Kettlebell: The kettlebell is a combination of aerobic and strength training and has been shown to burn about 20 calories per minute. 20 minutes of this exercise is an option for intense aerobic exercise during the shedding phase.

In addition to being a cardio exercise, 20 minutes of kettlebells is also an excellent way of strength training as well as coordination.

Other options include swimming, rowing, high-intensity interval training, jumping jacks, singles tennis. These can all be incorporated as a 20 minute plan.

Strength Training

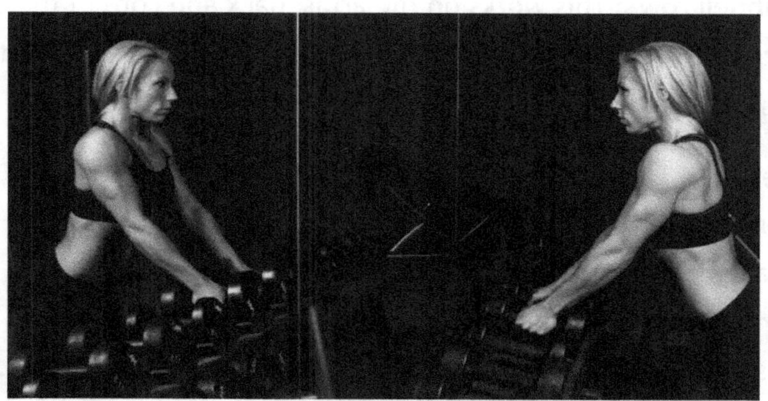

These sets of exercises work on multiple muscle groups at the same time and in addition to burning fat during the exercise, they keep the metabolism higher for a longer period of time after the workout has been completed. Strength training exercises increase the lean body mass which causes an increase in your metabolic rate, so helping with weight management. Having well-trained muscles also improves their ability to take up and use glucose which reduces the risk of diabetes. The other functions and targets of strength training include:

- ☐ Improved joint function
- ☐ Reduced risk of injury
- ☐ Increased bone density
- ☐ Improved cardiac function.

The strength exercises include:

Push-ups: The push-up is a simple exercise which works the upper body as well as the core. Five sets of 12 reps can be done while taking short breaks of 20-30s in between sets

Dumbbell rows: This works on the arms, back and core of the body. 3 sets of 15 reps on each hand daily helps to build strength in these parts.

Superman: This exercise is named after the comic character due to the resemblance the body bears to the super hero when he is in flight. While lying on the floor, 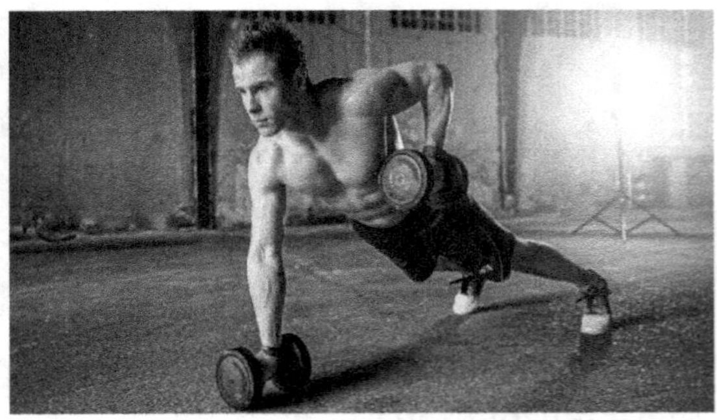 simultaneously raise your arms, legs, and chest off of the floor and hold this position for 2-3 seconds. Squeeze your lower back to get the best results from this exercise. Remember to exhale during this movement. Do 3 sets of 15 reps of this as well.

Other strength training exercises include bench presses, single-leg dumbbell row, squat to overhead press, pullups, and planks. These exercises can be carried out for periods of 20 minutes daily with breaks in between sets. Strength exercises have been shown to be the most effective in losing fat.

Stretching and Body Balancing Exercises

While stretching is not quite as effective as aerobic exercises and strength training exercises for burning fat, it still serves as an important means of burning fat. Stretching exercises help build up muscles which increases the metabolic rate and thus helps shed some fat as well. The stretching exercises can as well be targeted at various parts of the body as in the back, the neck, the abdomen, the thighs or waist to help lose fat in these specific areas.

Some simple stretch exercises include:

Cobra stretch: Lay flat on your stomach with hands under the shoulders at the same time ensuring that the thighs are parallel to each other and elbows placed near the body. Position the toes on the ground so as to act as supporters. One should start by stretching the arms outwards while making sure that the legs are high. Then one should move to a position where the body is 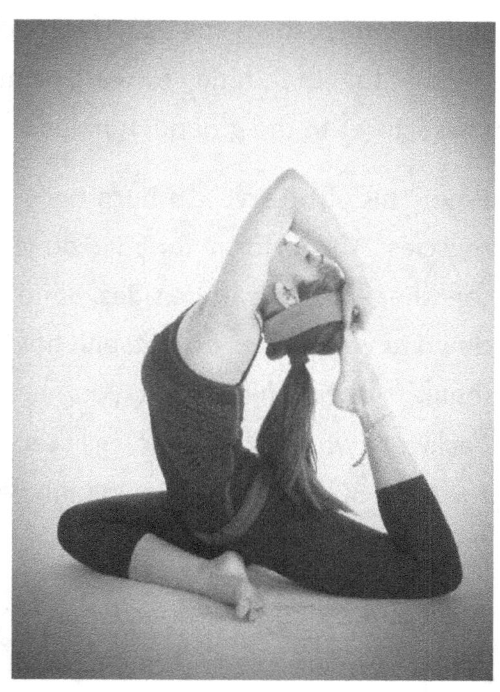 comfortable in the cobra position. While assuming the cobra yoga pose, relax the buttocks muscles while pressing the tailbone and pushing the shoulders together. Relax and hold the pose for 40 seconds to 2 minutes or as long as possible. Then slowly relax and stretch on the ground while taking in deep breaths. This helps to build up the abdominal muscles, burning some abdominal fat while giving the advantage of a more flexible spine and lengthening the shoulders, neck, abdomen and lungs. The cobra yoga stretch exercise is also effective in stimulating the digestive organs and also in alleviating stress.

Full body roll: To do this, stand tall and reach your arms upwards, then relax the arms and roll the spine down. Let your arms relax towards the floor. Keep the knees bent to protect your back. This can be done in sets of 15 seconds each after which you roll up and repeat.

Hip and inner thigh stretch: This is achieved by bringing the soles of the feet together, tilting forward from the hips and then bringing the chest closer to the ground. It helps to burn fat on the thighs.

Bow: This also serves to burn belly fat and tightens the abdominal muscles. To perform this, lie down prone with the legs straight together and arms at the sides. Bend your knees and reach your arms down to your ankles or feet, and hold the position for a few seconds. Inhale slowly while lifting your head, and then bend your head backward while lifting your legs as high as you can. Hold this position for 15 to 30 seconds while you inhale and exhale. Repeat 5 to 10 of this set while taking breaks in between.

The Board: is another effective means of burning the abdominal fat which many people find very difficult to lose. Stretch straight on the ground with your body weight placed on the hands and toes. Tighten your abdominal muscles and maintain this pose, ensuring that your body is straight and your hands are flat on the ground. Like the other stretch exercises, this can be maintained for 15 to 30 seconds and repeated about 5 times while taking short breaks in between each rep.

Other stretch exercises include the tree stretch, bridge, split squat, the chair hip stretch. The bridge and chair hip stretch help to burn fats in the back; the seal stretch, the good hip stretch and the track-star hip stretch help to lose some fat in the hips; planks, full body rolls, bow and board stretches burn belly fat; leg-ups, air cycling, table top crossovers are means to lose fat accumulated around the thighs.

Body balancing

training exercises have the added advantage of helping to keep you sure footed, improving posture and providing a much toned physique in addition to the main goal of losing fat. They work on multiple joints of the body over a range of motions to ensure that all muscle groups are put into use as opposed to the strength and resistance exercises which work on just one muscle group repetitively. A balance disk might be required for some of these exercises.

Balance training involves doing exercises that strengthen the muscles that help keep one upright, including the muscles of the legs and the core. As some of the exercises might entail closing the eyes and instead attempting to focus with the mind in order to maintain balance, these exercises help to keep the mind and body in sync and can even be used as relaxation techniques (yoga or tai chi)

Specific aims and actions of body balancing exercises include:

- Improving proprioception, the body's sense of its position in space
- Improves co-ordination
- Improves joint stability
- It improves the reaction time of the body in the event of an imminent fall
- Improves agility
- Increased balance improves long term health as it reduces the occurrence of falls and fractures in old age.

Examples include;

Single leg balance squat: Stand on one foot in front of a bench and squat till your buttocks touch the chair. Stand up using only the leg on which you were standing and repeat the exercise on the alternate leg.

Switch kicks: Stand with one foot placed on the balance disk. Bend the other knee in front of you and extend your arms to the sides. Tighten your core and perform a front kick with the bent leg. As soon as this foot completes the kick, slightly hinge forward at hips and swing the leg under body to carry out a back kick. Switch legs to complete set and keep on alternating the legs

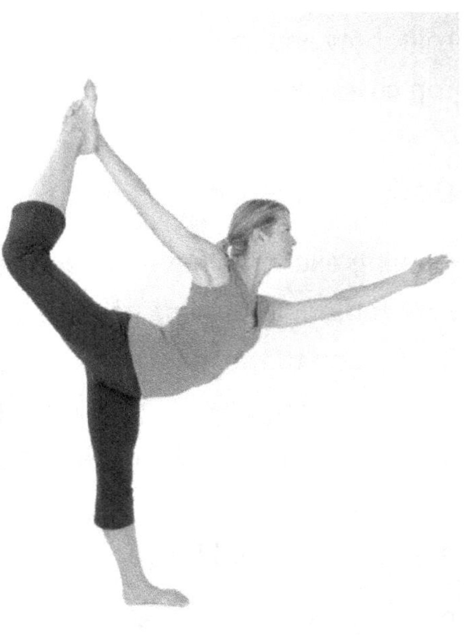

Seagull: Stand with one foot placed on the balance disk or aero pad. Bend other knee in front of you and extend the arms to the sides. Lean forward at hips, extending the bent leg behind you until the torso and leg are completely parallel with the floor. Pause and lower arms down in front of body with hands pointed to floor. Switch legs to complete set.

The stretching and balancing exercises can be allocated about ten minutes of the total work-out plans with breaks taken in between the sets as earlier advised for each of these exercises.

Creating a Personalised Plan

With the myriad options that exist in terms of exercises to embark upon, a key step towards using these exercises effectively is to create a plan that is best suited for you. To ensure that you have the right mix of the various forms of exercises, it is advisable to consider doing the following:

- Spend a larger amount of time on strength and resistance training than on stretching exercises as they are the most effective means of burning fat- this can be done such that there are two days of strength training alternating with one day of aerobic exercise if you decide to hit the gym.

- Ensure that you rest adequately in between sets of exercise to reduce the risk of injury and allow for better recovery by the muscle groups.

- Try to work on exercises which work on opposing groups of muscles alternately- for instance, exercises which pull on a muscle group can be alternated which those that require pushing on the next day, muscle groups can also be worked on alternate days by carrying our exercises that stretch the back today and those which work the front the next day. For example, a Day 1 workout might include goblet squats (which works on the lower front), rows (which exercise upper back), lateral lunges (works the bottom front), and push-ups (works the upper front), while Day 2 consists of dead lifts (work the lower back), overhead presses (work the upper front), step-ups (work the lower front), and lateral pulldowns (upper back).

- Take breaks when necessary and try as much as possible to enjoy the experience.

Holiday the Right Way

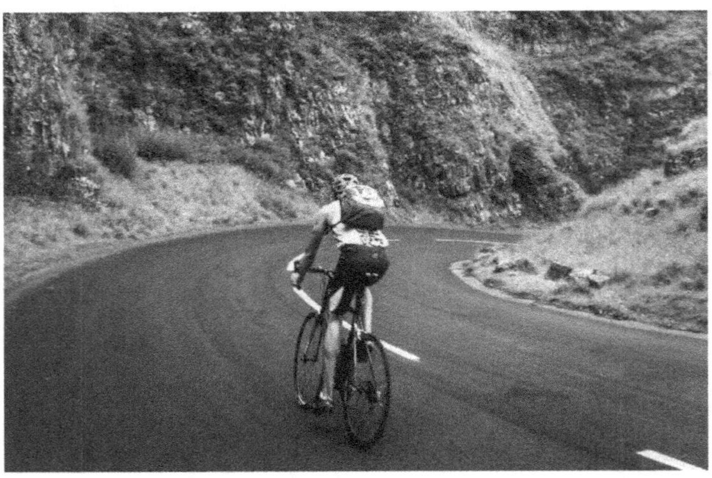

Incorporating your work out into vacations is also very important. A vacation is not the time to stay away from the healthy habits that have been built over a period of time but the time to keep up the good work that has been started. In addition to keeping up with regular exercise, it is pertinent to avoid eating excessively and feeding on junk foods which would counteract all the good work being put in.

The vacation is however supposed to be a fun period and a great way of losing fat and keeping fit while on vacation is to engage in fun activities which can double as workout routines. These activities include:

Beach walking: This has been shown to be a more effective means of losing weight than walking on the flat surface found everywhere normally.

Beach Volleyball: You have probably not had a vacation to talk about if you have not engaged in beach volleyball and while you are having fun, you are also losing some of the unwanted weight.

Cycling: While on vacation, cycling around town on a sightseeing journey is a tool to kill two birds with one stone.

Surfing: This is an intense exercise which has the advantage of working every muscle in the body and thus serving as a total body workout routine.

Football: Another fun means of aerobic exercise that equally works on various muscle groups.

Golf: While this is a low-intensity game, it can be made more effective by walking around the course instead of taking the ride around the golf course in which as much as 200 calories can be lost an hour.

Tennis: If played with a lot of fervour, tennis can be a very great workout plan, which can help burn as much as 500 calories in an hour.

Other fun activities such as **swimming, hiking, snorkeling** as well as many more sports can be great tools to keep in shape while on vacation.

PHASE 3:
MAINTENANCE PHASE

Like the name suggests, this is the phase in which one attempts to keep the body in the state that has been achieved by regular exercising. The maintenance phase is generally described as beginning after the first six months of exercise. In this phase, further improvements may not be very marked but the aim is to keep at the level of fitness that has already been acquired. The maintenance phase is one which requires long-term commitment and motivation in order not to stop working out. Keeping the body in its fit state after the initial intense workout can be achieved by:

Upping the cardio exercise

Focusing on cardio exercises will help to lose any fat that might remain while encouraging muscle gain and keeping the cardiovascular system even more healthy. Walking or jogging for 15-20 minutes per day is an effective form of aerobic exercise.

Working out for shorter periods and in a less intense manner:

Stretching and balance exercises are less intense exercises which are still useful to maintain the body in proper shape. The frequency of workout can also be reduced with attention shifted instead to full body workouts with compound movements that utilise a wider range of muscles.

A sample plan

Here is an example of a full body workout plan and is found to be effective when added to your daily routine.

Workout Regimen for weight maintainance	
Bench Press **3 sets of 10-12reps**	The muscles used here are triceps and pectoralis with deltoids. These are chest and upper arm muscles.
Bent Row **3 sets of 10-12reps**	This works the biceps and back muscles (rhomboids)
Military Press **2 sets of 10-12reps**	Involves backmuscles (rhomboids), arm and shoulder muscles (biceps, triceps, deltoids)
Squats **3 sets of 10-12reps**	Involves buttock muscles (gluteus), thigh muscles, hamstrings and quadriceps
Lunges **2 sets of 10-12reps**	Works same muscles in squats plus abdominal muscles and back muscles
Close Grip Bench Press **3 sets of 10-12reps**	This works on the triceps, a wider grip increases the work on your chest muscles.
Close Grip Barbell Curl **3 sets of10-12eps**	Involves biceps, brachialis and pectoralis muscles
Calf Raises **3 sets of 10-12reps**	Involves leg muscles (gastrocnemius, soleus, tibialisposterior).

The diet required to maintain the physique that has been built is slightly different from that used in building it in the first place. Instead of the high protein diets needed for the high metabolism rates in the initial phase, vitamins and minerals are essential to keep the muscles healthy.

Enrolling in sports within your local community can also serve to ensure that slacking off is less likely. Join a local tennis, volleyball, football or swimming club that meets on weekends. In deciding what sport to choose, it is advisable to go with one which you will most enjoy in order to ensure adherence.

RECORDING YOUR AWESOME PROGRESS

Recording the progress being made during the process of workout can be an important visual motivation that ensures that one continues to work on losing more weight. Various tools exist for keeping track of this progress including the use of fitness tracking applications or keeping a journal. Fitness applications have columns for inputting weight or abdominal girth measurements and then plot graphs to show how much progress is being made.

Keeping a journal is also a very effective way of tracking this process. Record the starting date and body weight as well as hip-waist ratios, record the exercise which you intend to embark upon for a particular day and mark them off once they have been completed. Input the specific, measurable, attainable and time specific goals which you have in mind. Obtain weekly measurements of weight and hip-waist ratios to see how much progress is being made. The weight can be used to calculate the Body Mass Index which provides an insight into just how much body fat is present. As simple as these steps may appear, they serve to provide much needed motivation for many individuals. Pictures can also serve as a means of recording the body transition that is going on and when significant progress is made can serve as reminders of what one used to look like. During this process, it is essential to keep working towards the SMART goal that has been set. Celebrate the little successes that you achieve weekly as they are thing to be proud of.

Finally, the reward system by which the brain operates is one which can be used to provide extra impetus to keep up the good work. These rewards do not have to be culinary and examples of such rewards that can be given once a weight loss goal is achieved include buying a new outfit, going on a vacation (at which you continue to work out), going to see a movie, attending a local sporting event, having a spa day or getting a facial. Keep yourself happy and enjoy the process of working out.

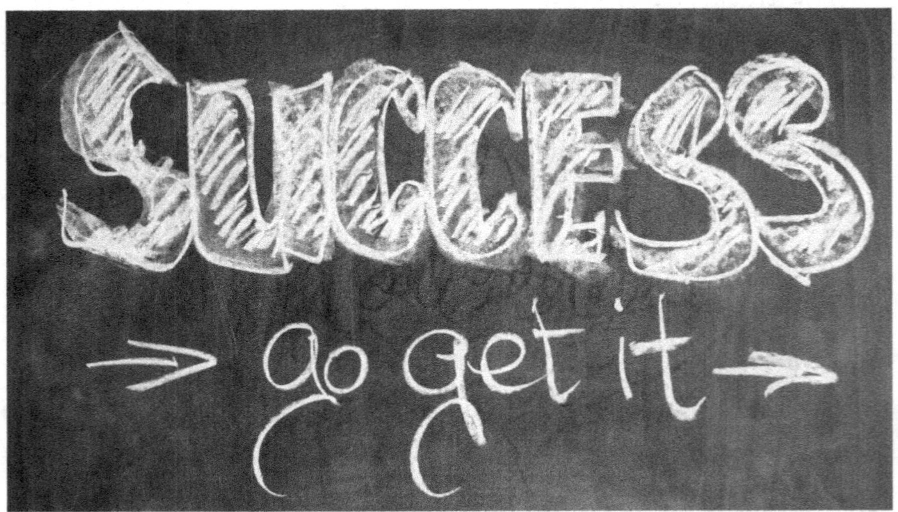

WORKOUT TRACKERS

Phase 1

	Time	Distance	Speed	Comments
Day 1				
Day 2				
Day 3				
Day 4				
Day 5				
Day 6				
Day 7				

Phase 2

	Week 1	Week 2	Week 3	Week 4	Week 5	Week 6	Week 7	Week 8
Cardio workouts								
Type of workout								
Time								
Distance								
Speed/intensity								
Comments								
Strength training								
Type of workout								
Time								
Intensity								
Comments								
Body stretching								
Type of workout								
Time								
Intensity/flexibility								
Comments								
Body Balancing								
Type of workout								
Time								
Intensity								
Comments								

Phase 3

Weight Maintenance Workout Sheet							
	Monday	Tuesday	Wednesday	Thursday	Friday	Saturday	Sunday
Bench Press **3 sets of** **10-12reps**							
Bent Row **3 sets of** **10-12reps**							
Military Press **2 sets of** **10-12reps**							
Squats **3 sets of** **10-12reps**							
Lunges **2 sets of** **10-12reps**							
Close Grip Bench Press **3 sets of** **10-12reps**							
Close Grip Barbell Curl **3 sets of** **10-12eps**							
Calf Raises **3 sets of** **10-12reps**							

PART 4

WEIGHT LOSS RECIPES

BREAKFAST

Egg wraps stuffed with chicken

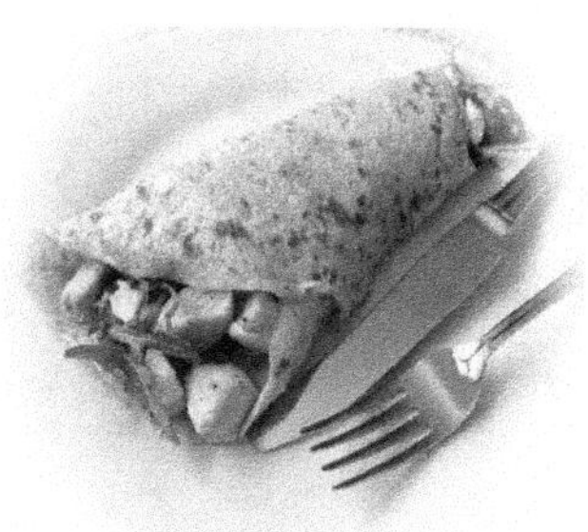

Ingredients:

- 3 egg whites
- ½ cup of chicken, cut into small pieces
- 1 tbsp of ginger paste
- ½ tbsp of garlic paste
- ¼ cup of arugula leaves
- 2 tbsp of chopped parsley
- ½ tbsp of freshly ground black pepper
- ½ tbsp of oregano
- ¼ tbsp of olive oil
- Salt to taste

Method:

1. In a bowl, add egg whites, chopped parsley, dried mint and salt.
2. Beat the mixture using an electric beater.
3. Add olive oil to a pan and this egg mixture.
4. Make a thin omelette.
5. In another pan, add chicken pieces, ginger paste, garlic paste, ground black pepper and salt.
6. Sauté the mixture for 6-9 min.
7. After that add arugula leaves and mix with the chicken mixture.
8. Arrange a small portion of chicken and arugula mixture on one side of omelette and roll it carefully.
9. Serve hot.

High protein sandwich

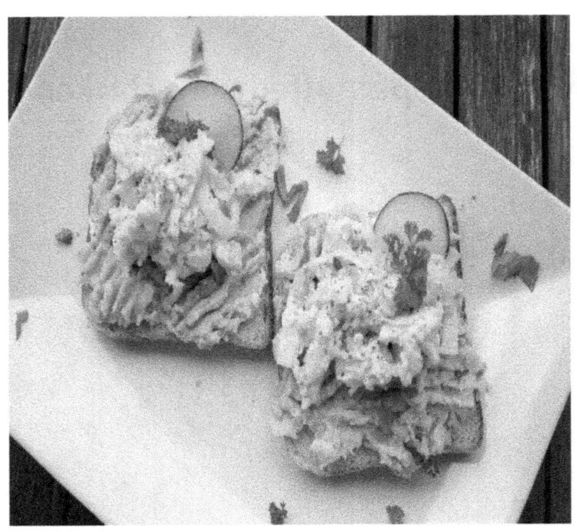

Ingredients:

- 2 slices of whole grain bread
- ¼ cup of avocado, mashed
- 3 eggs
- ½ tbsp of olive oil
- 1 tbsp of freshly ground black pepper
- Salt to taste

Method:

1. In a hot pan, add olive oil.
2. Add egg to the hot olive oil.
3. Add salt and black pepper to the egg mixture.
4. Give a thorough mix and turn off the heat.
5. In another bowl, add avocado, salt and pepper.
6. Mix them thoroughly and keep aside.
7. Spread the avocado mixture on whole grain bread slices.
8. Add scrambled egg on top and serve.

Omelette wrap with veggie stuff

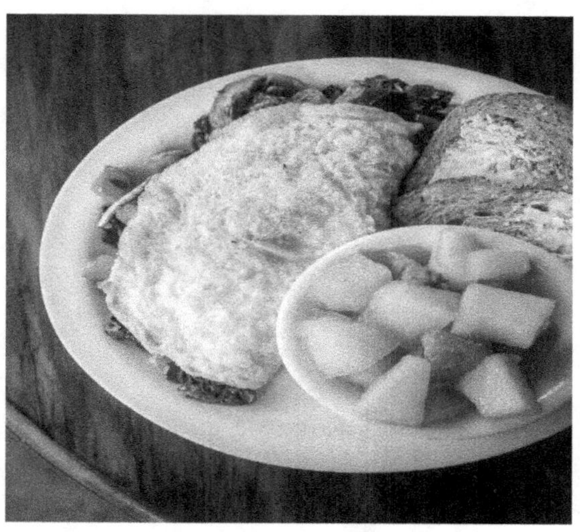

Ingredients:

- 2 eggs
- 1 tbsp of olive oil
- ¼ cup of kale leaves, chopped
- 1 tomato, chopped
- ½ tbsp of dill
- 1 tbsp of freshly ground black pepper
- A pinch of turmeric powder
- Salt to taste

Method:

1. In a bowl, add eggs, salt and turmeric powder.
2. Beat the mixture thoroughly and keep aside.
3. In a hot pan, add olive oil.
4. Add egg mixture to the pan.
5. Cook on both sides and keep aside.
6. In another bowl, add kale leaves, tomato, dill, freshly ground black pepper and salt.
7. Give a thorough mix.
8. Add this veggie mixture to the omelette and wrap it.
9. Serve.

Brown bread sandwich

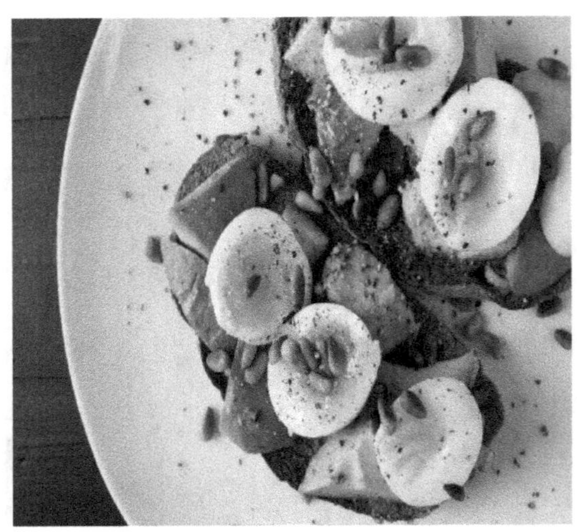

Ingredients:

- 2 slices of brown bread
- ½ cup of avocado, sliced
- 2-3 half boiled eggs, halved
- 2 tbsp of pine nuts, roasted
- 1 tbsp of freshly ground black pepper
- Salt to taste

Method:

1. In a bowl, add avocado, salt and ground pepper.
2. Give a thorough mix.
3. Add avocado mixture on the brown bread.
4. Add halved eggs on top of the avocado mixture.
5. Add pine nuts, pepper and a dash of salt.
6. Serve.

Italian style omellete

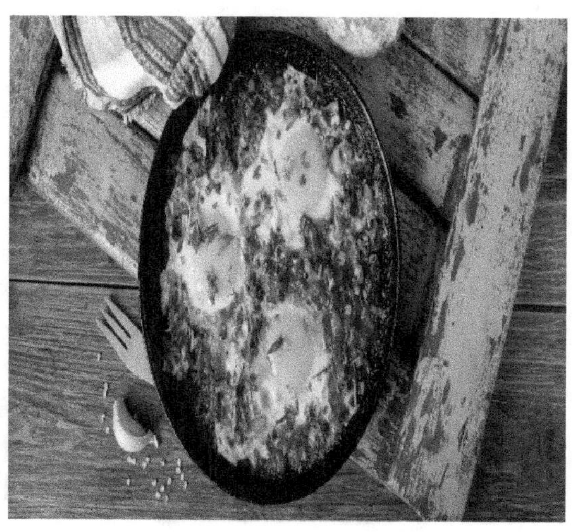

Ingredients:

- 3 eggs
- 1 cup of tomato puree
- 2 tbsp of garlic paste
- 1 tbsp of ginger paste
- 2 tbsp of coconut milk
- 2 tbsp of freshly ground white pepper
- Salt to taste

Method:

1. In a hot pan, add all the ingredients except eggs.
2. Bring the mixture to boil.
3. Add eggs to the tomato mixture.
4. Put the lid on and cook for another 5 min in medium heat.
5. Turn off the heat and serve.

Boiled chicken with green salad

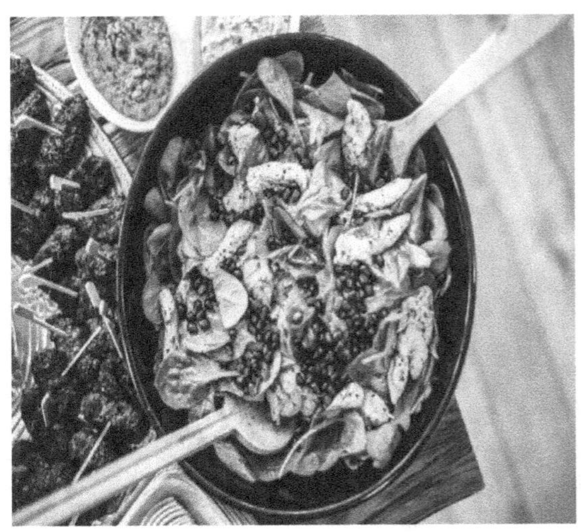

Ingredients:

- 1 cup of spinach leaves, cleaned
- ½ cup of chicken pieces, boiled
- ¼ cup of pomegranate seeds
- 1 tbsp of oregano
- ½ tbsp of lime juice
- 1 tbsp of freshly ground black pepper
- Salt to taste

Method:

1. Add all the ingredients to a bowl.
2. Give a thorough mix.
3. Serve.

Tasty omelette

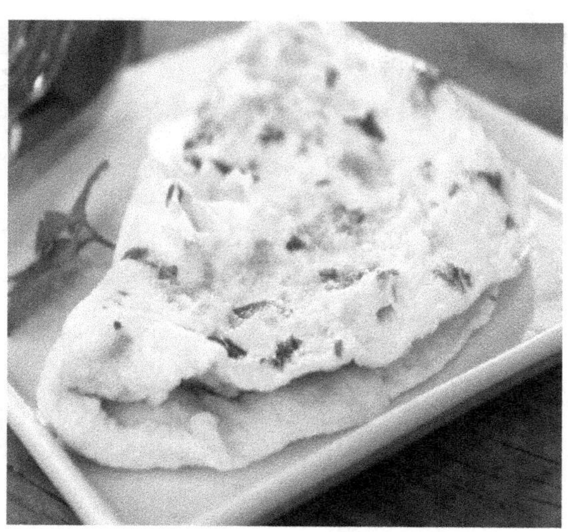

Ingredients:

- 3 eggs
- 1 tbsp of parsley, finely chopped
- 1 tbsp of lemon grass, chopped
- ½ tbsp of thyme
- ½ tbsp of turmeric powder
- 1 tbsp of freshly ground pepper
- 1 tbsp of olive oil
- Salt to taste

Method:

1. In a bowl, add all the ingredients except olive oil.
2. Give a thorough mix using an electric beater.
3. In a hot pan, add olive oil and egg mixture.
4. Cook at low heat with lid on.
5. Serve hot.

Egg & veggie frittata

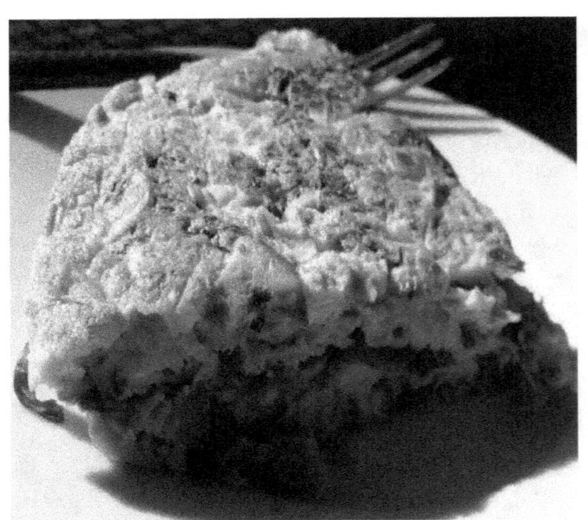

Ingredients:

- 4 egg white
- 3 egg yolks
- 1 tbsp of chopped mint
- ¼ cup of mushroom, chopped
- ¼ cup of kale, chopped
- 1 tbsp of freshly ground black pepper
- 1 tbsp of avocado oil
- Salt to taste

Method:

1. In a bowl, add all the ingredients, except avocado oil.
2. Beat the mixture using an electric beater.
3. In a hot pan, add avocado oil and egg mixture.
4. Cook at low heat with lid on for at least 5 min.
5. Turn sides of the frittata, so that the both sides cook evenly.
6. Serve hot.

Special egg sandwich

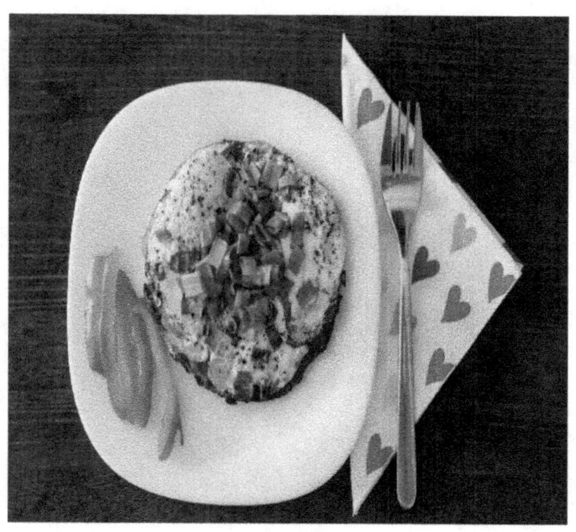

Ingredients:

- 1 slice of brown bread
- 2 eggs
- ½ tomato, sliced
- 1 tbsp of oregano
- ½ tbsp of freshly ground black pepper
- ¼ tbsp of olive oil
- Salt to taste

Method:

1. In a hot pan, add olive oil.
2. Add tomato slices, eggs, oregano, pepper and salt.
3. Cook for 2-3 min.
4. When the egg is cooked, transfer the egg to the brown bread.
5. Serve.

Garnish with onion leaves (optional).

Mushroom omelette

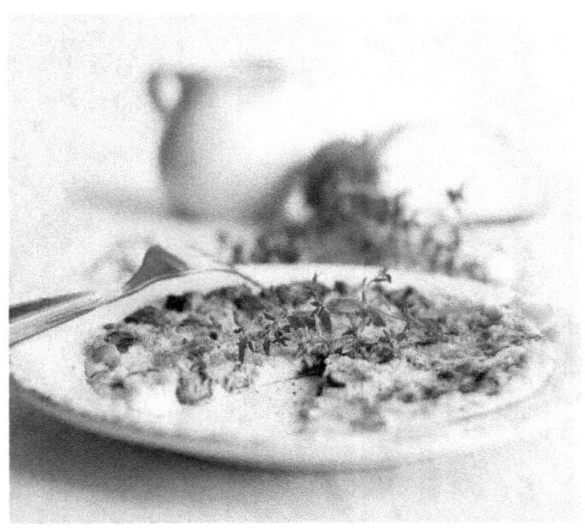

Ingredients:

- 3 eggs
- ¼ cup of mushroom, cut into small pieces
- ½ tbsp of thyme
- A pinch of turmeric powder
- 1 tbsp of freshly ground pepper
- 1 tbsp of olive oil
- Salt to taste

Method:

1. In a bowl, add all the ingredients except olive oil.
2. Give a thorough mix using an electric beater.
3. In a hot pan, add olive oil and egg mixture.
4. Cook at low heat with lid on.
5. Serve hot.

Fruits & veggie salad

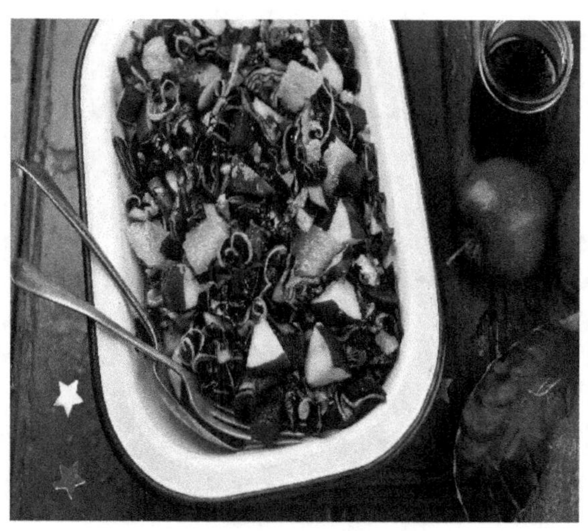

Ingredients:

- 1 cup of purple cabbage, cut into small pieces
- ½ cup of red apples, cut into small pieces
- ¼ cup of orange pieces
- ½ tbsp of balsamic vinegar
- 1 tbsp ground pepper
- 1 tbsp of olive oil
- Salt to taste

Method:

1. In a bowl, add all the ingredients.
2. Give a thorough mix and serve.

Greens & avocado mix

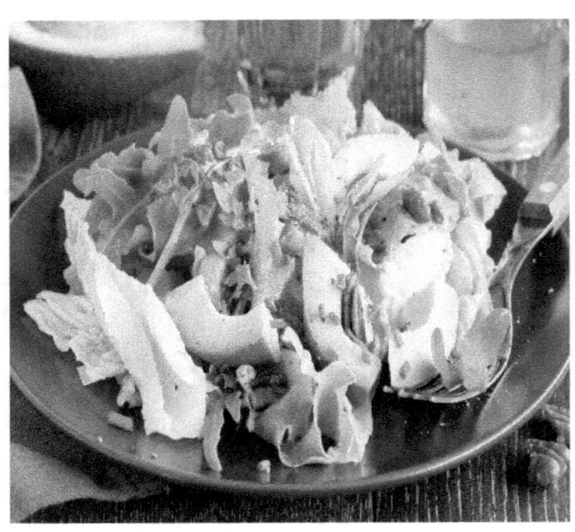

Ingredients:

- 1 cup of arugula leaves
- ¼ cup of green cabbage leaves, cut into small pieces
- ¼ cup of lettuce, cut into small pieces
- ¼ cup of avocado slices
- 1 tbsp of walnuts
- ½ tbsp of freshly ground pepper
- ¼ tbsp of lemon juice
- Salt to taste

Method:

1. In a bowl, add all the ingredients and give a thorough mix.
2. Serve.

LUNCH

Chicken Stew

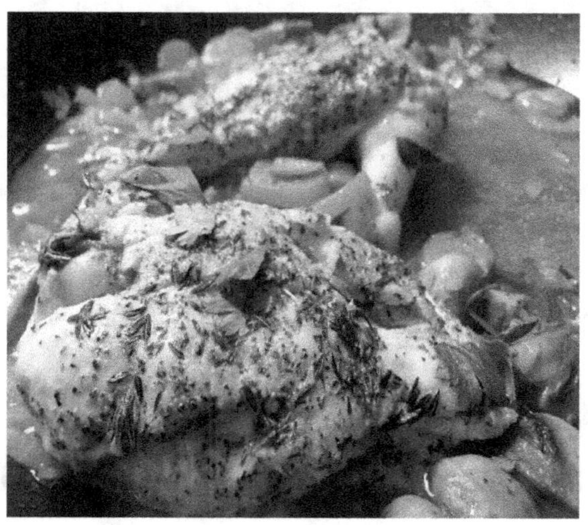

Ingredients:

- 200g of chicken
- ¼ cup of mushrooms
- 1 carrot, sliced
- 1 tbsp of dill
- 1 tbsp of oregano
- 1 tbsp of basil
- 1 tbsp of freshly ground black pepper
- ¼ cup of chicken stock water
- Salt to taste

Method:

1. In a pan, add all the ingredients and give a quick mix.
2. Cook in medium heat for 15 min.
3. Add small amount of water if necessary.
4. Serve hot.

Nuts coated steamed salmon

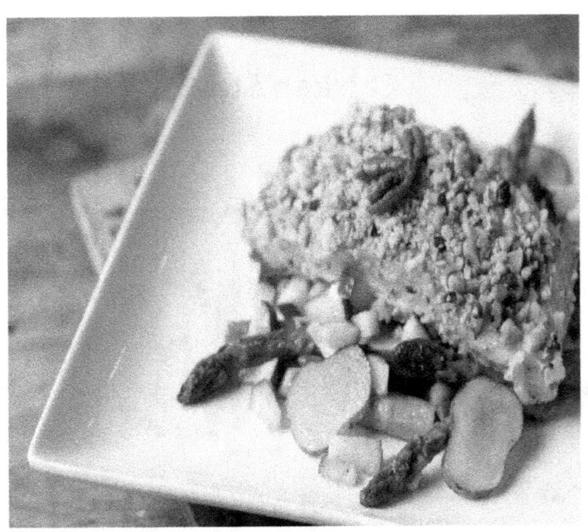

Ingredients:

- 100g of salmon
- 1 egg white
- 1 tbsp of lime juice
- ¼ tbsp of freshly ground white pepper
- ¼ cup of mixed nuts, roasted and crushed
- Salt to taste

Method:

1. In a bowl, add salmon, lime juice, pepper and salt.
2. Mix them thoroughly.
3. Allow the mixture to rest for 1 hour.
4. After 1 hour, dip the marinated salmon in egg white.
5. Roll it over on a plate full of crushed nuts.
6. Steam the nuts coated salmon for 10-15 min.
7. Serve hot.

Roasted chicken with oregano

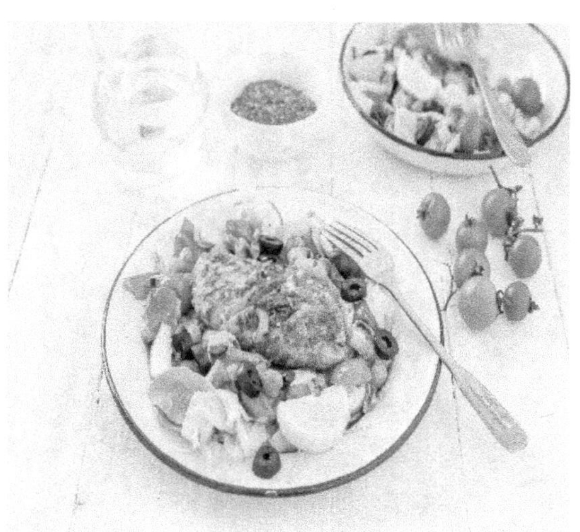

Ingredients:

- 150g of chicken breast
- 1 tbsp of garlic paste
- 1 tbsp of ginger paste
- ½ tbsp of freshly ground black pepper
- 1 tbsp of oregano
- ½ tbsp of apple cider vinegar
- Salt to taste

Method:

1. In a bowl, add all the ingredients.
2. Give a thorough mix.
3. Allow the chicken breast to marinate for 2 hours.
4. After 2 hours, transfer the chicken breast to a baking tray.
5. Bake at 180C for 35-40 min.
6. Serve hot.

Baked salmon in tamarind sauce

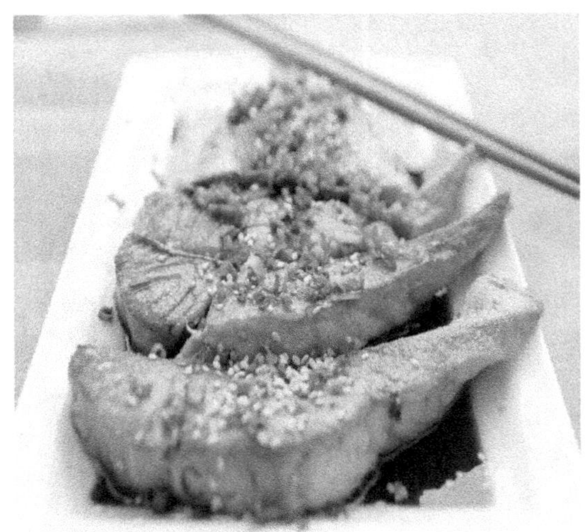

Ingredients:

- 2-3 slices of salmon
- 1 tbsp of lemon juice
- ½ tbsp of ginger paste
- ¼ tbsp of garlic paste
- A pinch of turmeric powder
- 2 tbsp of tamarind paste
- 2 tbsp of freshly ground black pepper
- Salt to taste

Method:

1. In a bowl, add all the ingredients.
2. Mix them thoroughly and allow the mixture to rest for 2 hours.
3. After 2 hours, transfer the sockeye salmon pieces to a baking tray.
4. Bake at 180C for 25-30 min.
5. Serve hot.

Toasted broccoli and chicken pieces

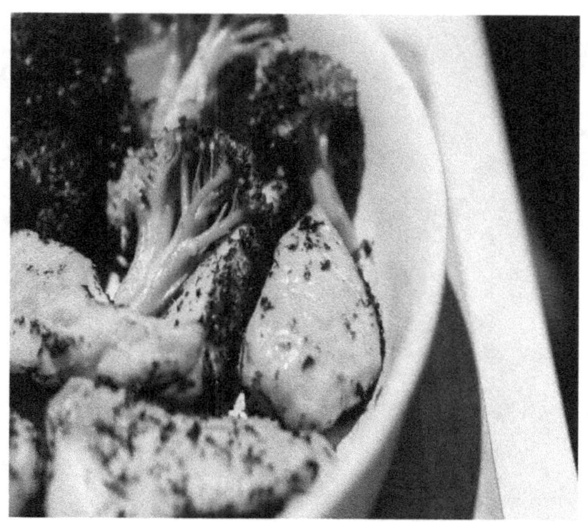

Ingredients:

- 1 cup of chicken pieces, cooked
- 1 cup of broccoli florets
- 1 tbsp of dried mint
- 1 tbsp of oregano
- 1 tbsp of freshly ground black pepper
- 1 tbsp of lime juice
- ½ tbsp of olive oil
- 1 tbsp of garlic powder
- Salt to taste

Method:

1. In a pan, add all the ingredients, except lime juice.
2. Give a quick mix.
3. Sauté in medium heat for 10 min.
4. Add small amount of water if necessary.
5. Serve hot.

Chicken roulette

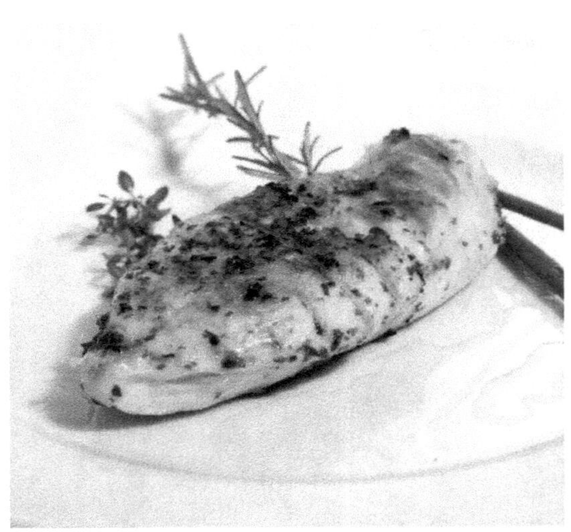

Ingredients:

- ½ chicken breast slice
- ¼ cup of cottage cheese
- 1 cup of finely chopped celery leaves
- 2 tbsp of parsley leaves, chopped
- 1 tbsp of lemongrass
- 1 tbsp of dill
- ½ tbsp of lime juice
- 1 tbsp of freshly ground black pepper
- Salt to taste

Method:

1. In a bowl, add cottage cheese, celery leaves, parsley leaves, ground pepper and salt.
2. Mix them thoroughly and keep aside.
3. In another bowl, add chicken slice, dill, lemongrass, lime juice, black pepper and salt.
4. Mix them thoroughly and allow the mixture to rest for 1 hour.
5. Add cottage cheese mixture and roll the chicken pieces.
6. Tie the chicken pieces with a thread to hold the cottage mixture in place.
7. Bake at 180C for 35 min.
8. Serve hot.

Roasted chicken breast

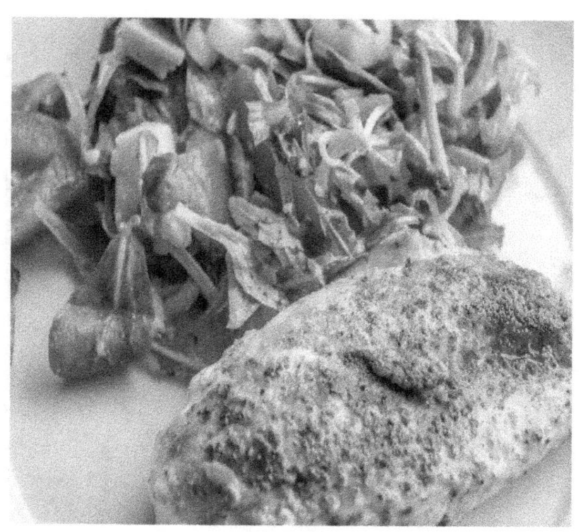

Ingredients:

- 250g of chicken breast
- 1 tbsp of ginger powder
- 1 tbsp of garlic powder
- 1 tbsp of orange juice
- 1 tbsp of freshly ground white pepper
- Salt to taste

Method:

1. In a bowl, add all of the ingredients in a bowl.
2. Mix the chicken piece with the spices thoroughly.
3. Allow the chicken piece to rest for 2 hours in a refrigerator.
4. Transfer the marinated chicken breast piece to a baking tray.
5. Bake at 180C for 30 min.
6. Serve hot.

Beef stuffed mushroom

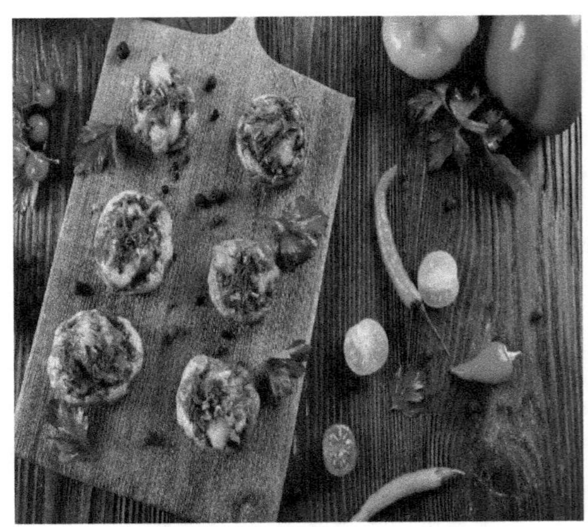

Ingredients:

- 4-6 Mushroom caps
- ½ cup of minced beef
- 1 tbsp of cottage cheese
- 1tbsp of chopped mint leaves
- 2 tbsp of chopped red bell pepper
- 1 tbsp of freshly ground black pepper
- Salt to taste

Method:

1. Mix all the ingredients in a bowl, except mushroom caps.
2. Stuff the mixture to the mushroom caps.
3. Transfer the mushroom caps to a baking tray.
4. Bake at 180C for 20 min.
5. Serve hot.

Toasted veggies and chicken

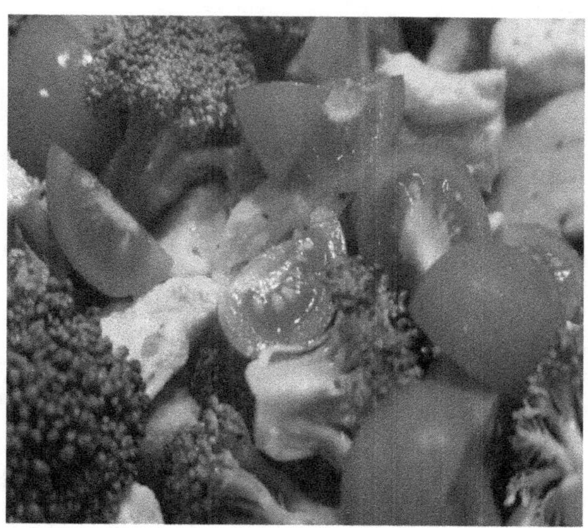

Ingredients:

- 1 cup of broccoli florets, steamed
- ½ cup of cherry tomatoes, halved
- 1 cup of chicken breast, cut into small pieces and steamed
- 1 tbsp of ginger, chopped
- ¼ tbsp of garlic, chopped
- 1 tbsp of oregano
- ¼ tbsp of olive oil
- 1 tbsp of freshly ground black pepper
- Salt to taste

Method:

1. In a hot pan, add olive oil and all the ingredients, except cherry tomatoes
2. Toss the mixture for 5 min.
3. Allow the mixture to cool.
4. Add halved cherry tomatoes to the mixture.
5. Mix them thoroughly and serve.

Baked tuna and veggie salad

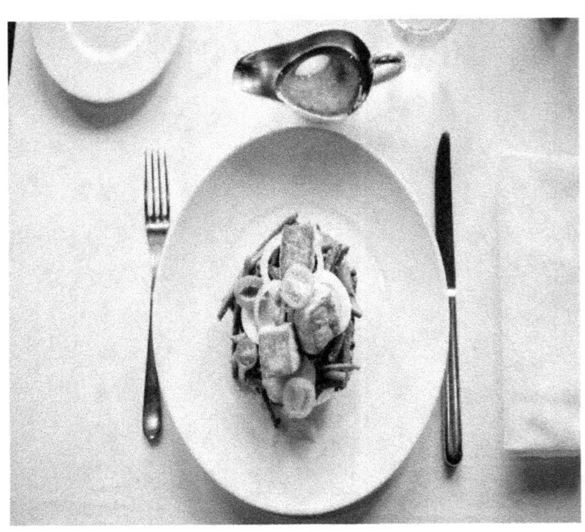

Ingredients:

- 1 cup of tuna chunks
- ½ cup of beans, steamed
- 6 cherry tomatoes, halved
- 1 boiled egg, halved
- ½ cup of red bell pepper sliced
- 1 tbsp of olive oil
- ¼ tbsp of freshly ground pepper
- Salt

Method:

1. In a bowl, add tuna chunks, freshly ground pepper and salt.
2. Mix them thoroughly allow them to marinate for 20 min.
3. After 20 min, transfer the tuna to a baking tray.
4. Bake at 150C for 20 min.
5. Add baked tuna with steamed beans, egg, cherry tomatoes, bell pepper and salt.
6. Give a gentle mix.
7. Serve.

Roasted chicken in honey marinade

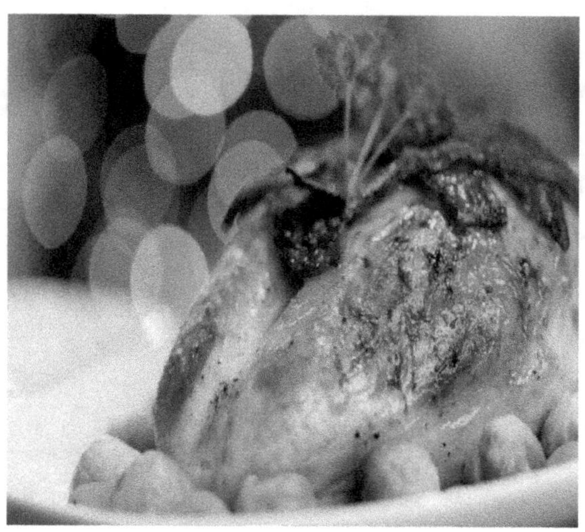

Ingredients:

- 1 small chicken breast
- 1 tbsp of ginger paste
- 2 tbsp of garlic paste
- ½ tbsp of thyme
- ¼ tbsp of oregano
- ¼ tbsp of cinnamon powder
- 1 tbsp of olive oil
- 1 tbsp of freshly ground pepper
- Salt to taste

Method:

1. In a bowl, add chicken breast, ginger paste, garlic paste, thyme, oregano, cinnamon powder, olive oil and salt.
2. Mix them thoroughly and marinate for 2 hours in a refrigerator.
3. After 2 hours, transfer the marinated chicken breast to a baking tray.
4. Bake at 180C for 45 min.
5. Serve hot.

Herbs infused roasted pork

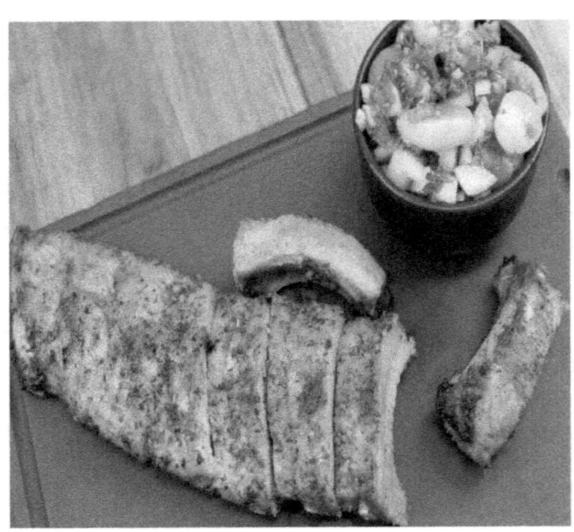

Ingredients:

- 150g of trimmed pork
- 1 tbsp of freshly ground black pepper
- 1 tbsp of orange juice
- ½ tbsp of dill
- ¼ tbsp of dried mint, crushed
- ¼ tbsp of oregano
- Salt to taste

Method:

1. In a bowl, add all the ingredients.
2. Mix them thoroughly.
3. Allow the mixture to marinate for 2 hours.
4. After 2 hours, transfer the marinated pork to a baking tray.
5. Bake at 180C for 45 min.
6. Serve hot with fresh veggie salad.

DINNER

Chicken and zucchini noodles

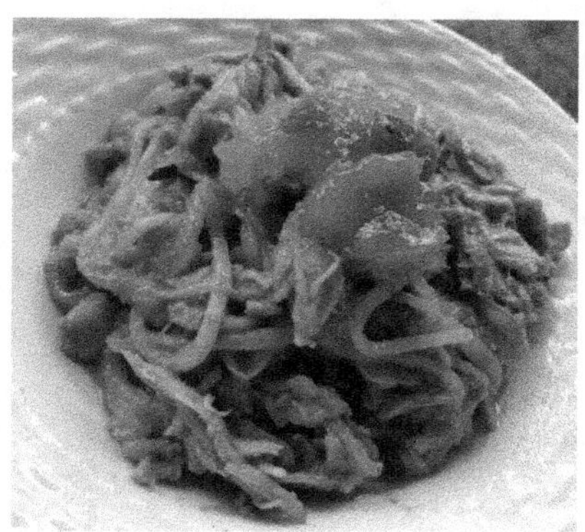

Ingredients:

- 1 cup of Spiralised zucchini
- 125g of chicken, cut into small pieces
- ½ onion, cut into thin slices
- 1 tomato, chopped
- 1 tbsp of tomato paste
- 1 tbsp of paprika powder
- 1 tbsp of ginger paste
- 1 tbsp of garlic paste
- 1 tbsp of freshly ground black pepper
- 1 tbsp of avocado oil
- Salt to taste

Method:

1. In a hot pan, add olive oil.
2. Add garlic paste, ginger paste, chicken pieces and salt.
3. Sauté them for 10 min.
4. Add tomato paste and chopped tomato.
5. Sauté them for another 2 min.
6. Put the lid on and cook for another 3 min.
7. After the chicken is cooked, add spiralised zucchini to the mixture.
8. Add paprika powder and sliced onions to the chicken mixture.
9. Serve.

Pumpkin & chicken soup

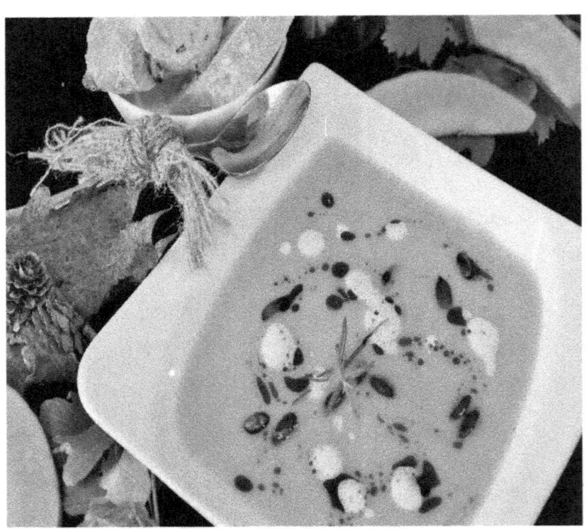

Ingredients:

- 1 cup of pumpkin, cubed
- 100g of chicken breast
- 1 cup of chicken stock water
- 2 garlic clove, chopped
- A pinch of turmeric powder
- Salt to taste

Method:

1. In a soup vessel, add all the ingredients.
2. Mix them thoroughly.
3. Put the lid on and bring the mixture to boil for 15 min.
4. Allow the mixture to cool.
5. After that, blend the mixture using a blender.
6. Serve.

Lemon infused chicken

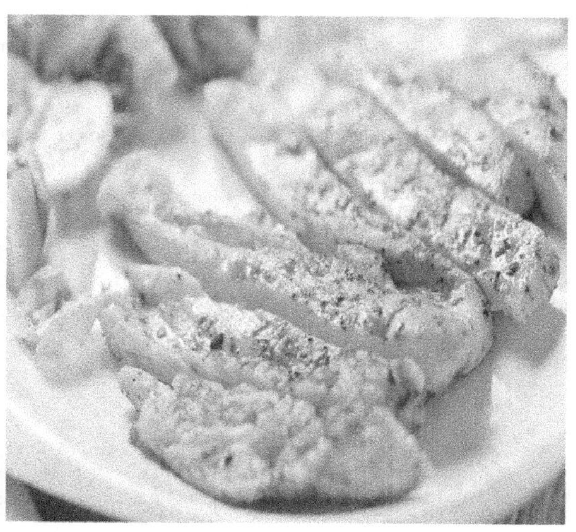

Ingredients:

- 125g of chicken breast, cut into strips
- 3 tbsp of lemon juice
- 1 tbsp of freshly ground black pepper
- ½ tbsp of oregano
- Salt to taste

Method:

1. Add all the ingredients to a bowl.
2. Mix them thoroughly and allow the mixture to rest for 30 min.
3. After 30 min, transfer the marinated chicken breast strips to a baking tray.
4. Bake at 175C for 30 min.
5. Serve hot.

Brussels sprout casserole

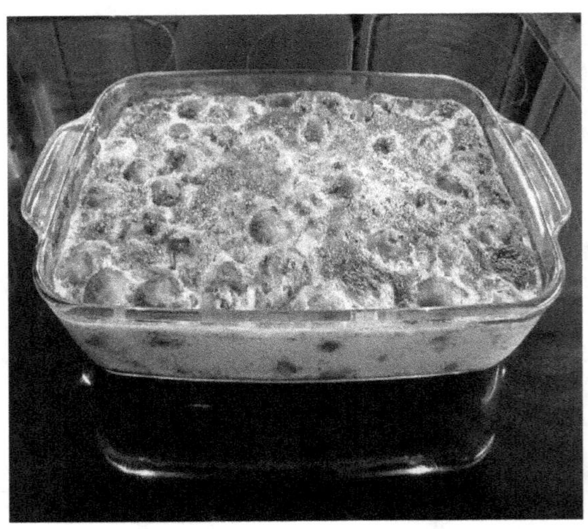

Ingredients:

- 100g of Brussels sprouts
- 5 egg whites
- ¼ cup of almond milk
- ½ cup of roasted chicken, cut into small pieces
- ½ tbsp of garlic powder
- ½ tbsp of freshly ground white pepper
- ½ tbsp of dried sage
- Salt to taste

Method:

1. Add all ingredients to a bowl.
2. Mix them thoroughly.
3. Transfer the content to a casserole baking tray.
4. Bake the casserole at 180C for 30 min.
5. Serve hot.

Baked salmon piece in lemon

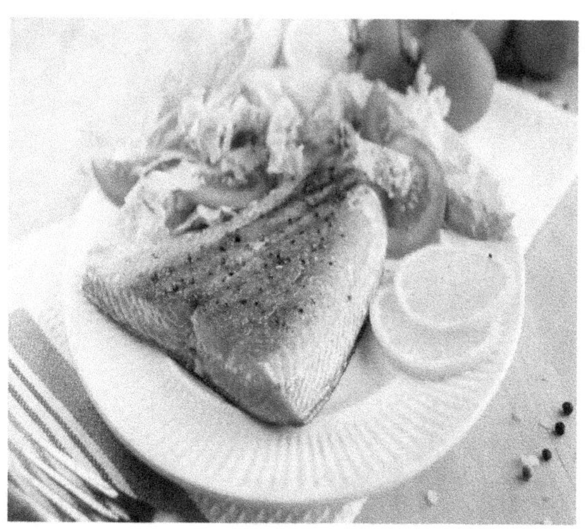

Ingredients:

- 150g of salmon
- 3 tbsp of lemon juice
- 1 tbsp of freshly ground black pepper
- 1 tbsp of oregano
- ½ tbsp of dried mint
- 1 tbsp of olive oil
- Salt to taste

Method:

1. Add all the ingredients to a bowl.
2. Mix them thoroughly and allow the mixture to rest for at least 30 minutes.
3. After 30 min, transfer the salmon piece to a baking tray.
4. Bake at 175C for 20 min.
5. Serve hot.

Orange infused trout baked

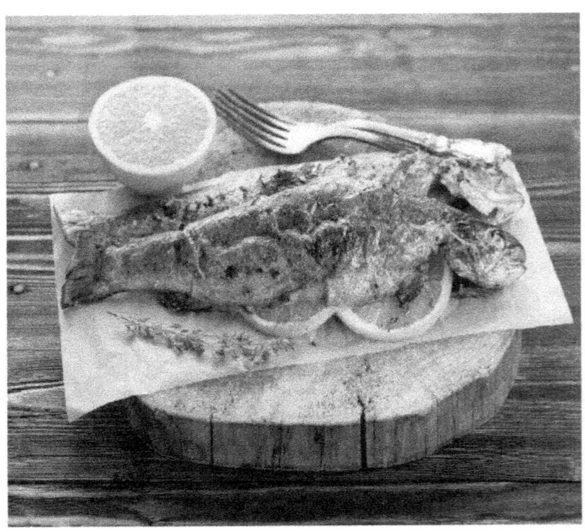

Ingredients:

- 300g of trout fish cleaned
- 1 tbsp of apple cider vinegar
- ½ tbsp of mint powder
- ¼ tbsp of olive oil
- ¼ tbsp of turmeric powder
- 3 tbsp of orange juice
- 1 tbsp of freshly ground black pepper
- Salt to taste

Method:

1. In a bowl, add all the ingredients.
2. Give a thorough mix and keep aside to rest for 45 min.
3. After 45 min, transfer the marinated fish to a baking tray.
4. Bake at 180C for 25 min.
5. Serve hot.

Beef casserole

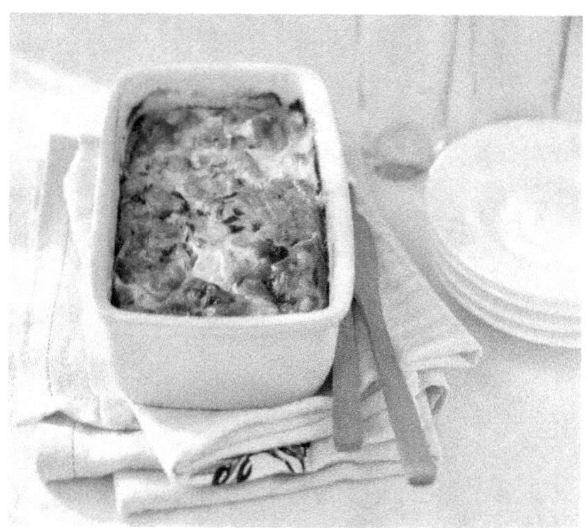

Ingredients:

- 200g of beef minced meat
- 1 cup of carrot, cubes (small cubes)
- ¼ cup of red bell pepper, cubes (small cubes)
- ¼ cup of chopped kale
- 3 egg whites
- 1 tbsp of thyme, dried
- ½ tbsp of turmeric powder
- ½ tbsp of freshly ground pepper
- Salt to taste

Method:

1. In a bowl, add all the ingredients and give a thorough mix.
2. Transfer the content to a casserole backing tray.
3. Pre-heat the oven at 180C for 4 min.
4. Bake the casserole at 180C for 30 min.
5. Serve hot.

Spicy chicken roast

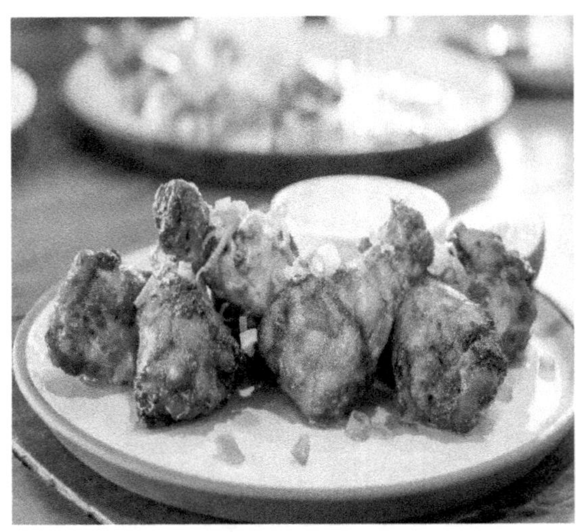

Ingredients:

- 200g of chicken pieces
- 1 tbsp of tamarind paste
- ½ tbsp of paprika powder
- ¼ tbsp of cinnamon powder
- ½ tbsp of mint powder
- ¼ tbsp of ginger paste
- ½ tbsp of garlic paste
- ¼ tbsp of balsamic vinegar
- Salt to taste

Method:

1. In a bowl, add all the ingredients and mix it thoroughly.
2. Allow the mixture to rest in the refrigerator for 2 hours.
3. After 2 hours, transfer the content to a baking tray.
4. Pre-heat the oven at 180C for 5 min.
5. Roast the chicken pieces at 180C for 35-40 min.
6. Serve hot.

Egg and bell pepper casserole

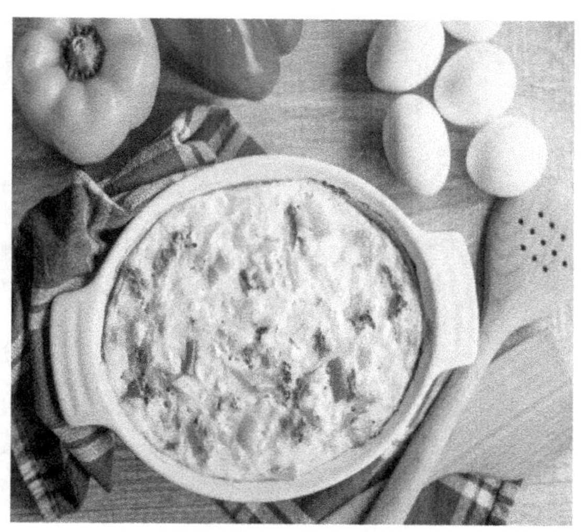

Ingredients:

- 250g of chicken pieces
- 6 eggs
- ½ cup of cottage cheese
- 1 cup of red bell pepper, diced
- ½ cup of green bell pepper, diced
- 1 tbsp of garlic, chopped
- ½ tbsp of freshly ground black pepper
- ¼ cup of broccoli florets
- Salt to taste

Method:

1. In a bowl, add all the ingredients and give a thorough mix.
2. Transfer the content to a casserole tray.
3. Bake at 180C for 35 min.
4. Serve hot.

Grilled chicken breast

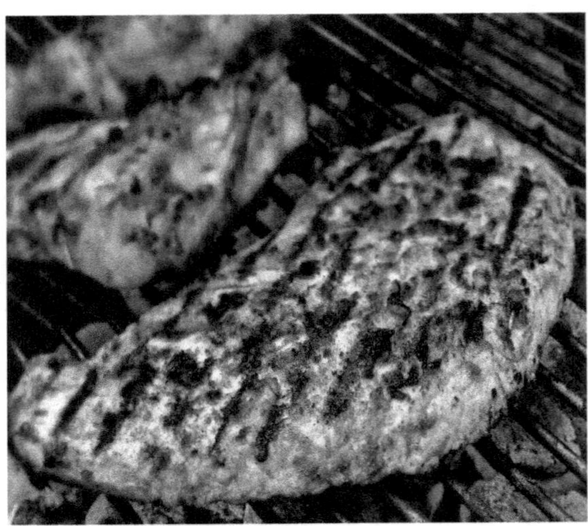

Ingredients:

- 250g of chicken breast
- 1 tbsp of ginger paste
- 1 tbsp of garlic paste
- ½ tbsp of paprika powder
- 2 tbsp of tomato paste
- 2 tbsp of balsamic vinegar
- 1 tbsp of freshly ground black pepper
- Salt to taste

Method:

1. In a bowl, add all the ingredients and mix them thoroughly.
2. Allow the chicken pieces to marinate for at least 2 hours.
3. After 2 hours, turn on the electric griller and place the marinated chicken pieces.
4. Grill on both sides every 4 min, until the meat is cooked.
5. Serve hot.

Green soup

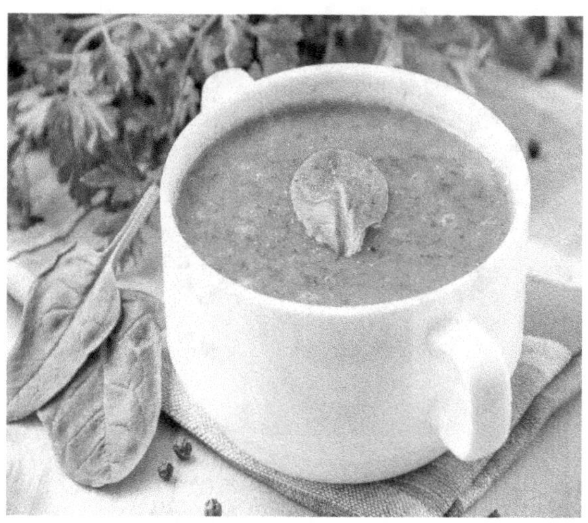

Ingredients:

- 1 cup of spinach leaves, chopped
- 1 cup of kale leaves, chopped
- 1 cup of chicken stock water
- 1 tbsp of freshly ground pepper
- ½ tbsp of dill
- 1 tbsp of lemon juice
- Salt to taste

Method:

1. In a vessel, add all the ingredients except lemon juice and dill.
2. Bring the mixture to boil for at least 10 min with lid on.
3. After 10 min, turn off the heat and allow the mixture to cool.
4. Add the green mixture to a blender and blend them thoroughly.
5. Add lemon juice, dill and salt (if required).
6. Serve hot.

Beef and veggie roulette

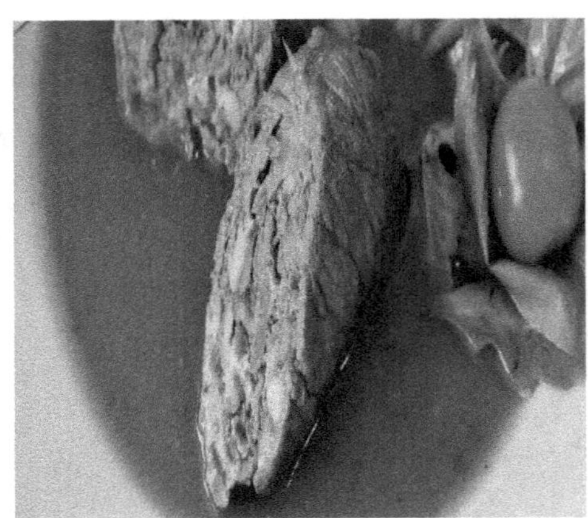

Ingredients:

- 1 (125g) thin slice of beef meat
- ½ cup carrot, cut into small pieces
- ¼ cup of beans, cut into small pieces
- 100g of beef meat, cut into small pieces
- 1 tbsp of garlic paste
- ½ tbsp of ginger paste
- 1 tbsp of freshly ground black pepper
- ½ tbsp of apple cider vinegar
- Salt to taste

Method:

1. In a bowl, add all the ingredients, except beef slice.
2. Mix them thoroughly and keep aside.
3. Arrange the beef slice on a board and add the mixture on one side of slice and roll the meat tightly.
4. If you need, use a long toothpick to secure the roll.
5. Transfer the roll to a baking tray.
6. Bake at 180C for 35-45 min.
7. Serve hot with tomato sauce.

SNACK

Beef cutlet

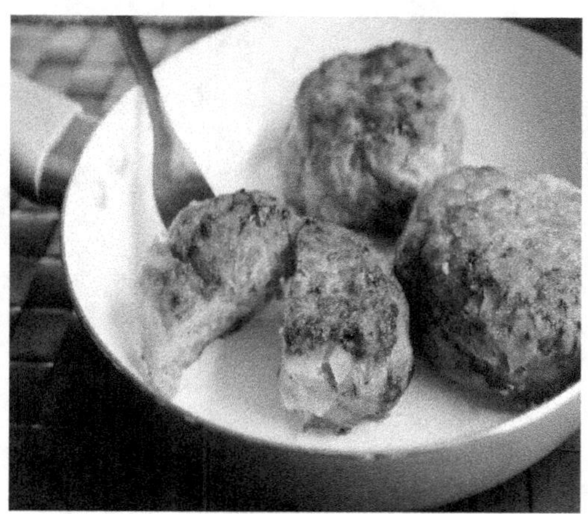

Ingredients:

- 1 cup of minced beef
- 1 tbsp of garlic, chopped
- 1 tbsp of ginger, chopped
- 1 tbsp of freshly ground black pepper
- ½ onion, finely chopped
- Salt to taste

Method:

1. In a bowl, add all the ingredients.
2. Mix them thoroughly into a soft dough.
3. Divide equal portions and make small balls or any desired shape.
4. Transfer the cutlets to a baking tray.
5. Bake at 180C for 20-25 min.
6. Serve hot.

Baked anchovies in garlic

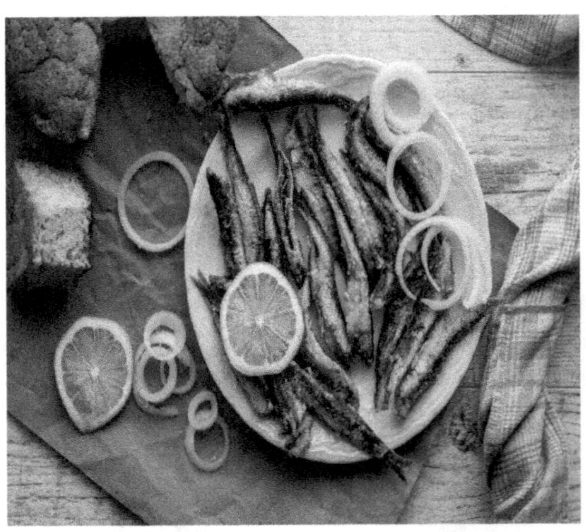

Ingredients:

- 150 g of anchovies, cleaned
- 1 tbsp of turmeric powder
- 3 tbsp of garlic powder
- ½ tbsp of lemon juice
- ½ tbsp of olive oil
- Salt to taste

Method:

1. Add all ingredients to a bowl.
2. Mix them thoroughly.
3. Allow the mixture to rest for 30 min.
4. After 30 min, transfer the anchovies to a baking tray.
5. Bake at 175C for 25 min.
6. Serve hot.

Fish cutlet

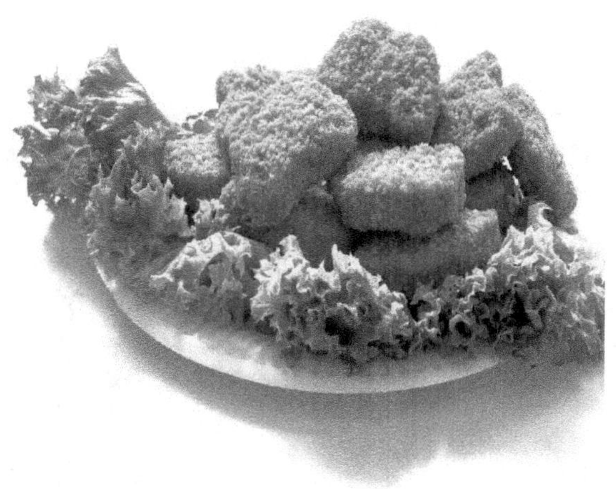

Ingredients:

- 100g of tuna, canned
- 1 tbsp of red onion, chopped
- ½ tbsp of parsley, chopped
- 1 egg
- 1 tbsp of lime juice
- 1 tbsp of freshly ground black pepper
- 1 cup of breadcrumbs
- Salt to taste

Method:

1. In a bowl, add all of the ingredients except egg and breadcrumbs.
2. Mix them thoroughly and make a soft dough.
3. Divide into equal portions and cut them into the desired shape.
4. Add the cutlet into the egg mixture and roll it into breadcrumbs.
5. Arrange the cutlets on a baking tray.
6. Bake at 180C for 20 min.
7. Serve hot.

Crispy baked tuna

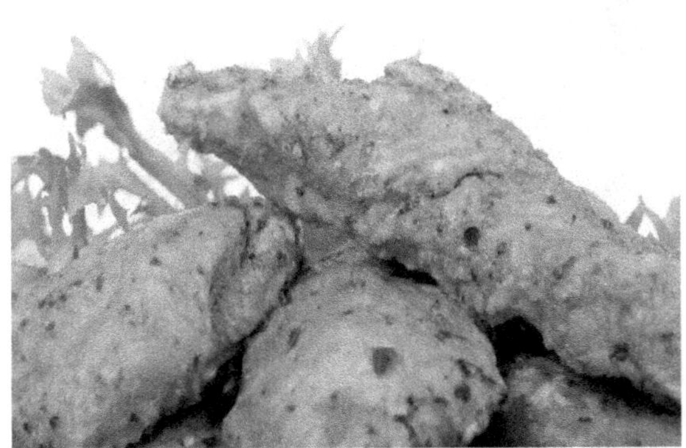

Ingredients:

- 150g of tuna pieces, canned
- 1 egg
- 1 tbsp of almond milk
- 1 tbsp of paprika powder
- 1 tbsp of garlic paste
- 1 tbsp of ginger paste
- ¼ tbsp of freshly ground black pepper
- Salt to taste

Method:

1. In a bowl, add all the ingredients except tuna pieces.
2. Beat the mixture using a hand whisk.
3. Add the tuna pieces to the egg mixture.
4. Transfer the egg coated tuna pieces to the baking tray.
5. Bake at 180C for 25 min.
6. Serve hot.

DETOX RECIPES

Baby spinach & parsley smoothie

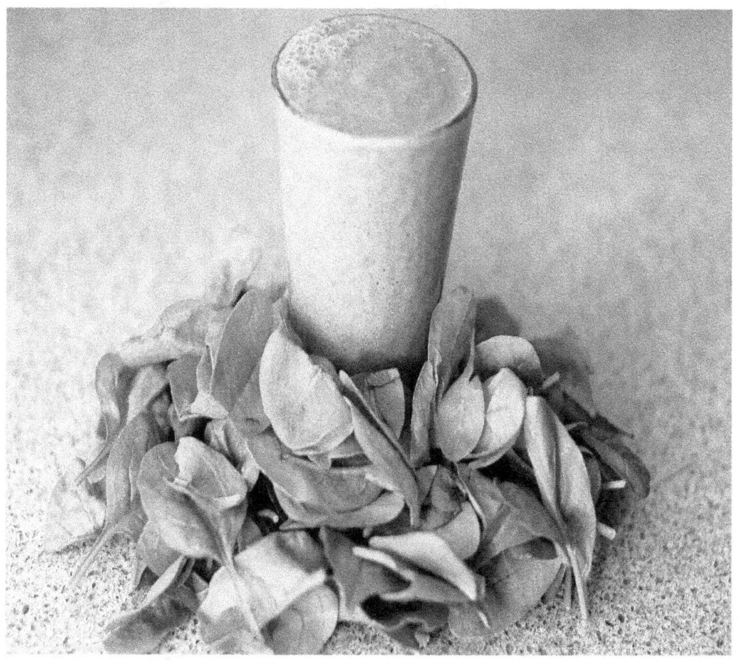

Ingredients:

- 1 cup of baby spinach, cleaned
- ½ cup of parsley, cleaned
- 1 tbsp of lime juice
- ½ cup of water

Method:

1. In a blender, add all the ingredients.
2. Blend the mixture thoroughly.
3. Serve chilled.

Fruits & veggie smoothie

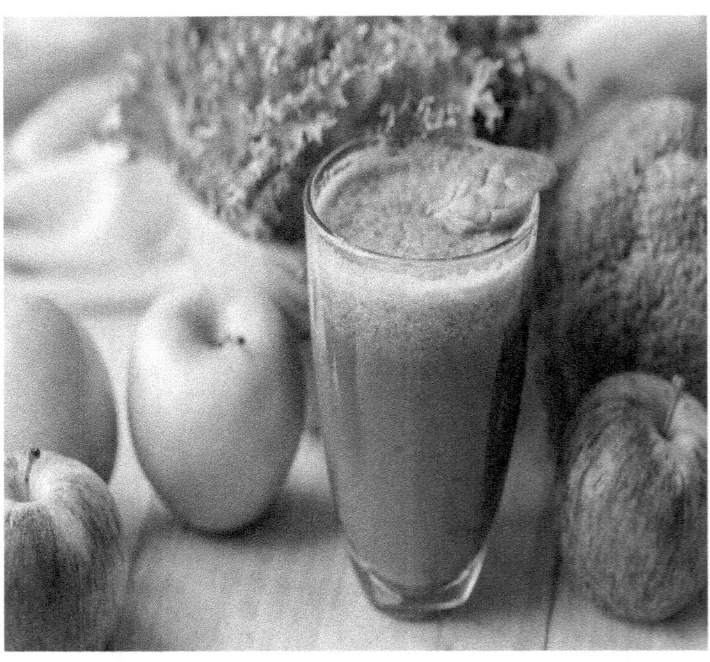

Ingredients:

- 1 green apple, cleaned and cubed
- 1 cup of kale, cleaned
- ¼ cup of broccoli, cleaned
- ½ red apple, cleaned and cubed
- 1 cup of water

Method:

1. In a blender, add all the ingredients.
2. Blend the mixture thoroughly.
3. Serve chilled.

Calories 92.5   **Serves 1**

Passion fruit smoothie

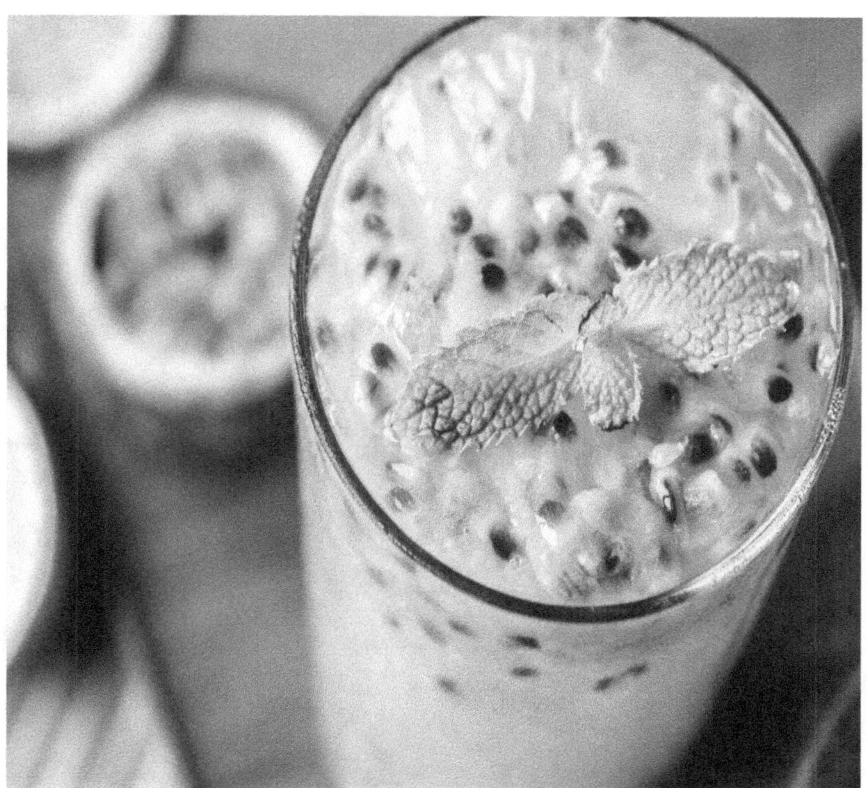

Ingredients:

- 1 cup of passion fruit pulp
- ½ tbsp of honey
- ½ cup of ice cubes
- ¼ cup of water

Method:

1. In a blender, add all the ingredients.
2. Blend the mixture thoroughly.
3. Serve chilled.

Nectarine with kale smoothie

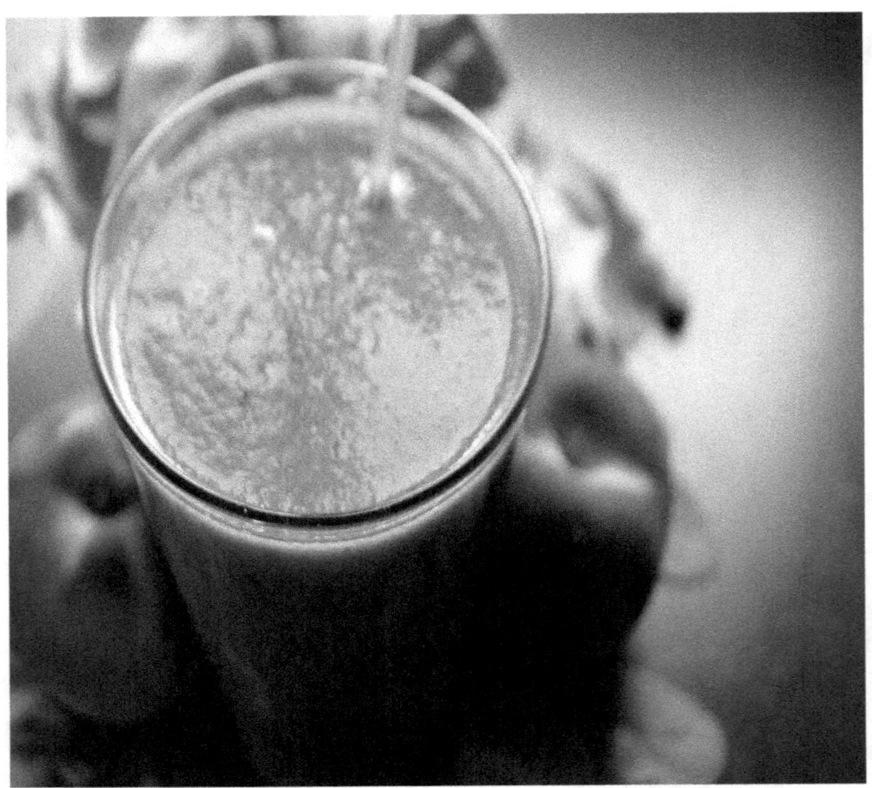

Ingredients:

- 1 cup of kale, cleaned
- 2 medium size nectarine, seeded and cubed
- ½ cup of water

Method:

1. In a blender, add all the ingredients.
2. Blend the mixture thoroughly.
3. Serve chilled.

Spinach & banana smoothie

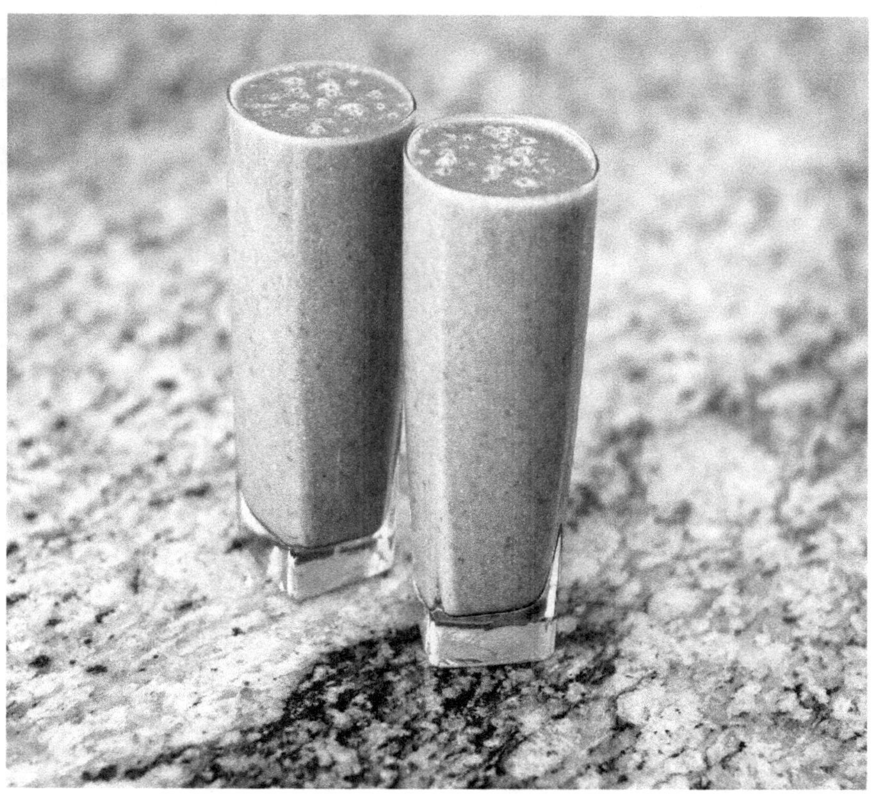

Ingredients:

- 1 cup of spinach leaves, cleaned and chopped
- 2 medium size banana, sliced
- 1 cup of water

Method:

1. In a blender, add all the ingredients.
2. Blend the mixture thoroughly.
3. Serve chilled.

Star fruit & spinach smoothie

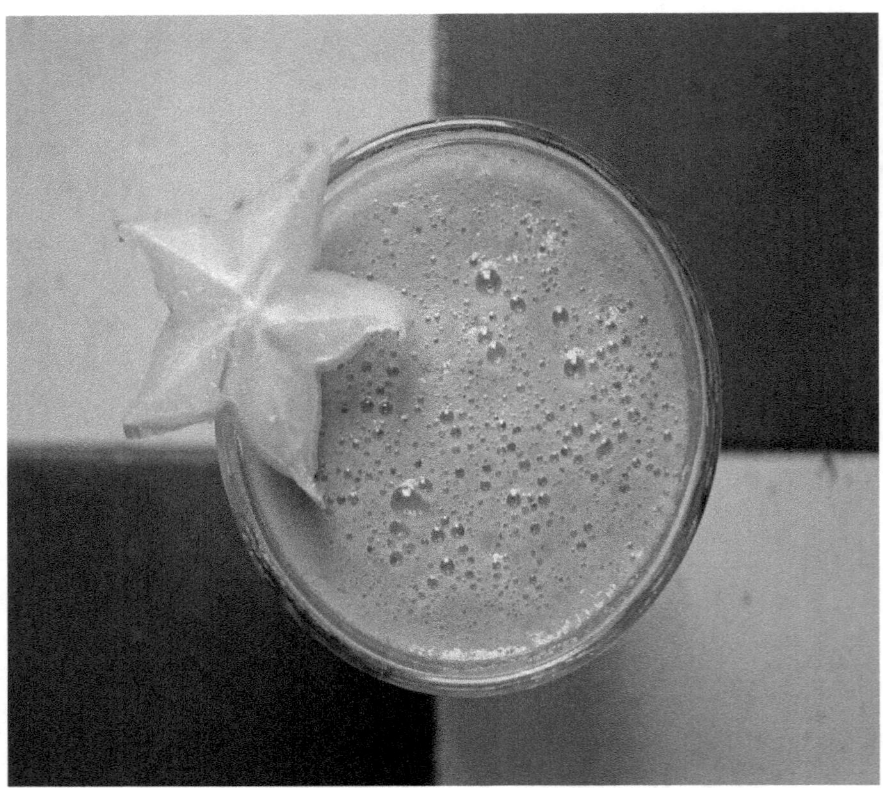

Ingredients:

- 1 cup of star fruit, sliced
- ½ cup of baby spinach leaves, cleaned
- 1 cup of water

Method:

1. In a blender, add all the ingredients.
2. Blend the mixture thoroughly.
3. Serve chilled.

Mint & kale smoothie

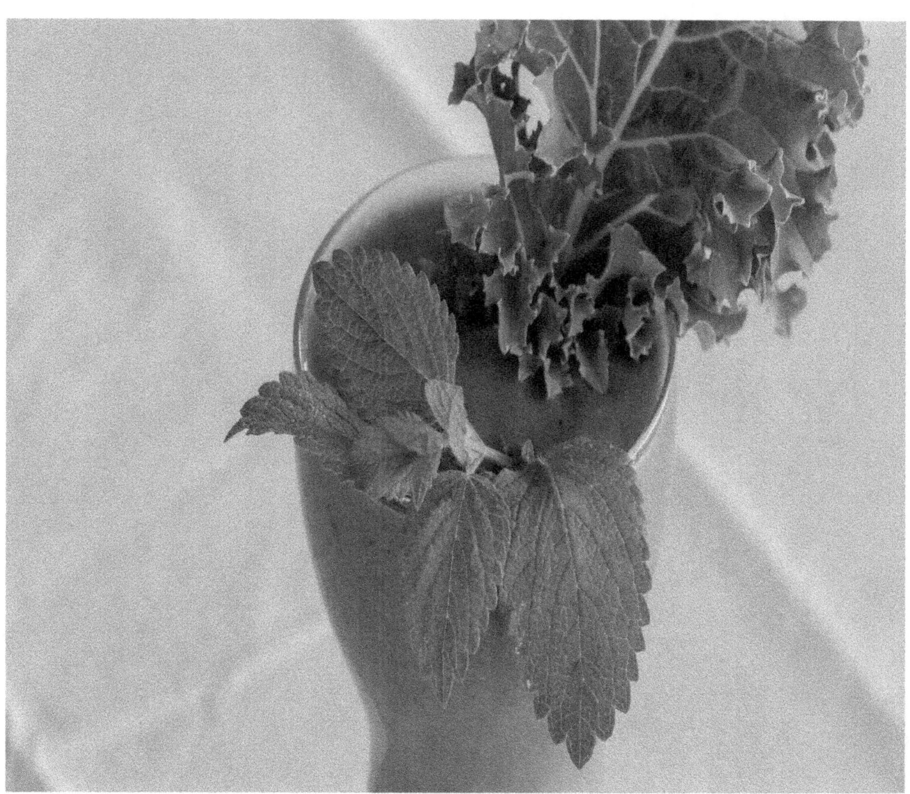

Ingredients:

- 1 cup of kale, cleaned
- ½ cup of mint leaves, cleaned
- 1 tbsp of lemon juice
- ½ cup of water

Method:

1. In a blender, add all the ingredients.
2. Blend the mixture thoroughly.
3. Serve chilled.

Calories 92.5

Serves 1

Kiwi with mint smoothie

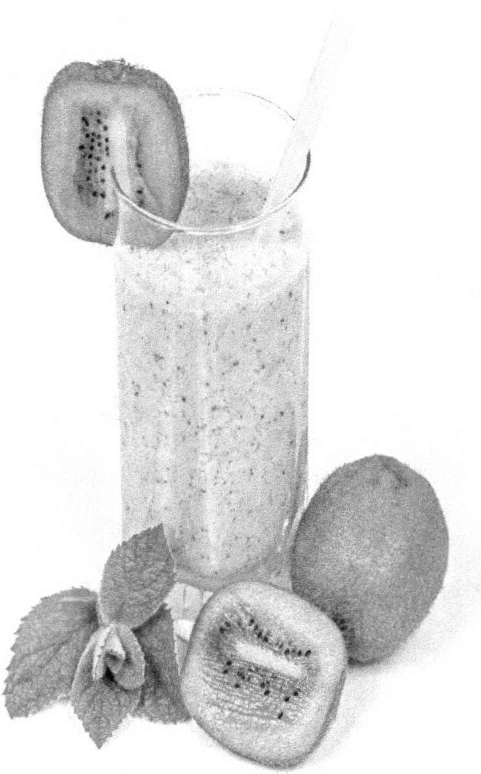

Ingredients:

- 1 cup of kiwi, cleaned and sliced
- 2 tbsp of mint leaves, chopped
- ½ cup of water

Method:

1. In a blender, add all the ingredients.
2. Blend the mixture thoroughly.
3. Serve chilled.

Apple & orange smoothie

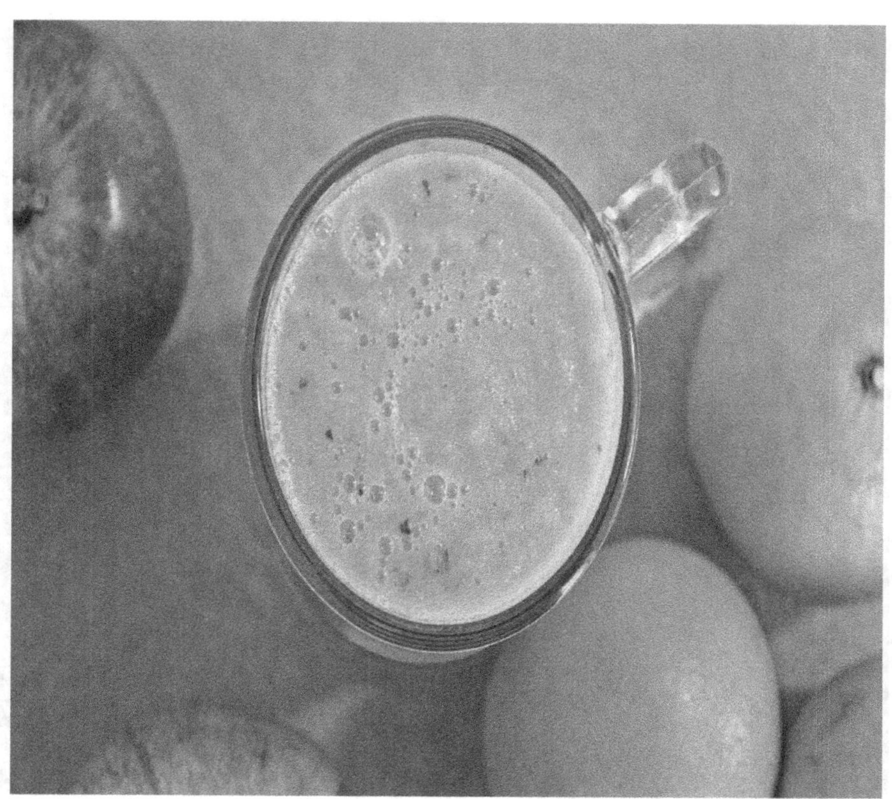

Ingredients:

- 1 red apple, seeded and sliced
- 1 orange, juiced
- 1 tbsp of honey
- ½ cup of water

Method:

1. In a blender, add all the ingredients.
2. Blend the mixture thoroughly.
3. Serve chilled.

Apricots & ginger smoothie

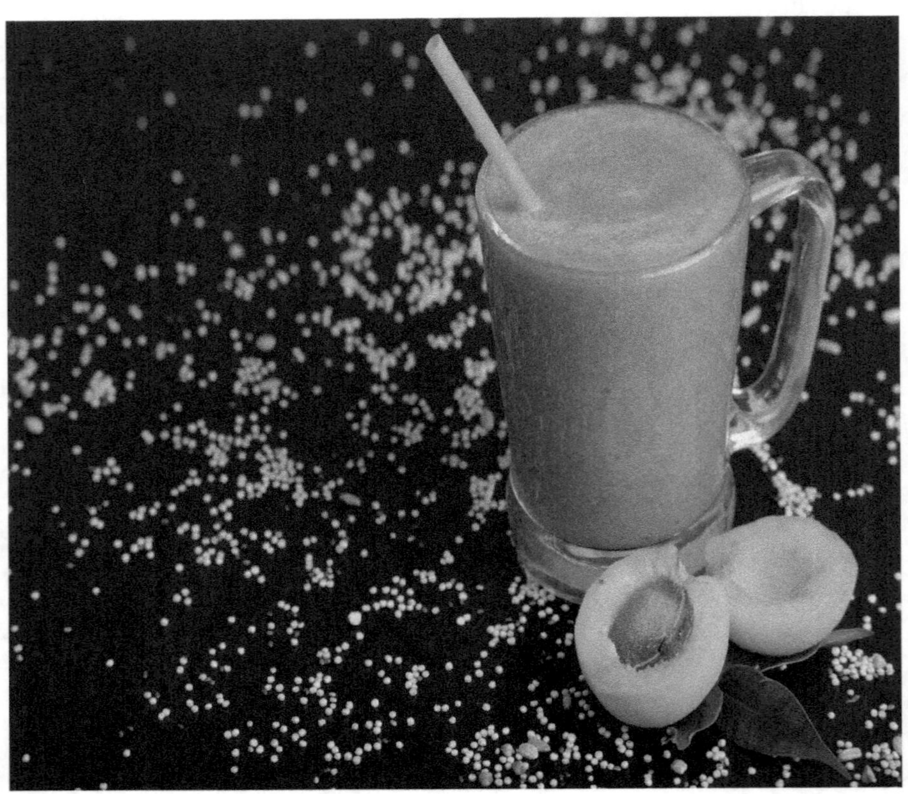

Ingredients:

- ½ cup of apricots
- 1 tbsp of ginger, chopped
- 1 cup of water
- ¼ tbsp of honey

Method:

1. In a blender, add all the ingredients.
2. Blend the mixture thoroughly.
3. Serve chilled.

Plums & blueberry smoothie

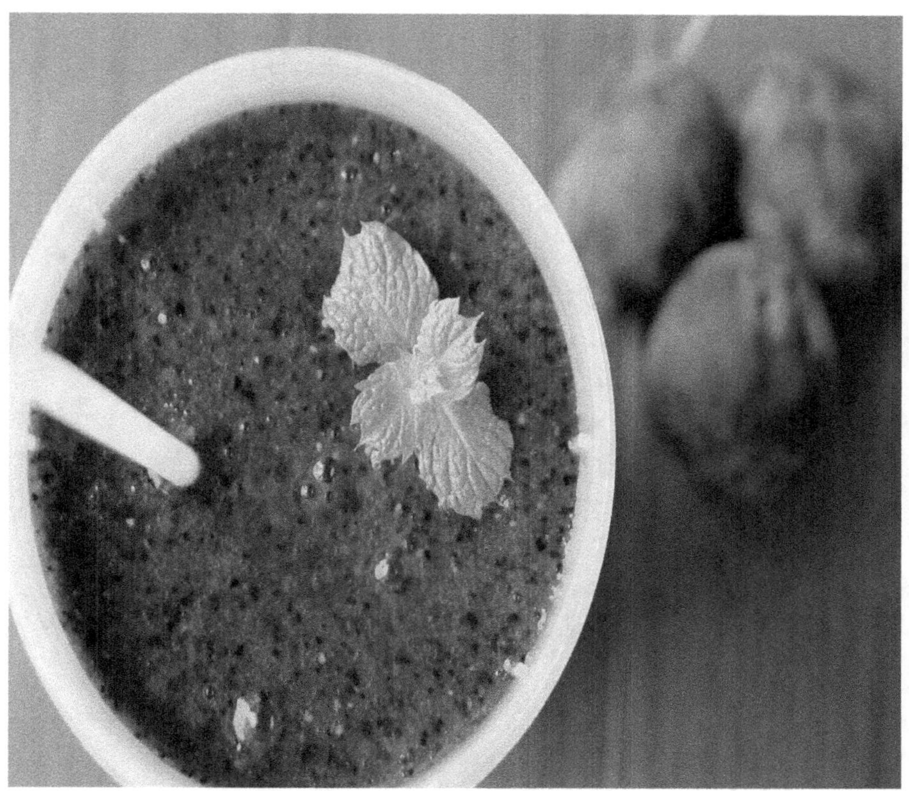

Ingredients:

- 1 cup of plums, seeded and sliced
- 1 cup of blueberry, cleaned
- 1 cup of water

Method:

1. In a blender, add all the ingredients.
2. Blend the mixture thoroughly.
3. Serve chilled.

Mango smoothie

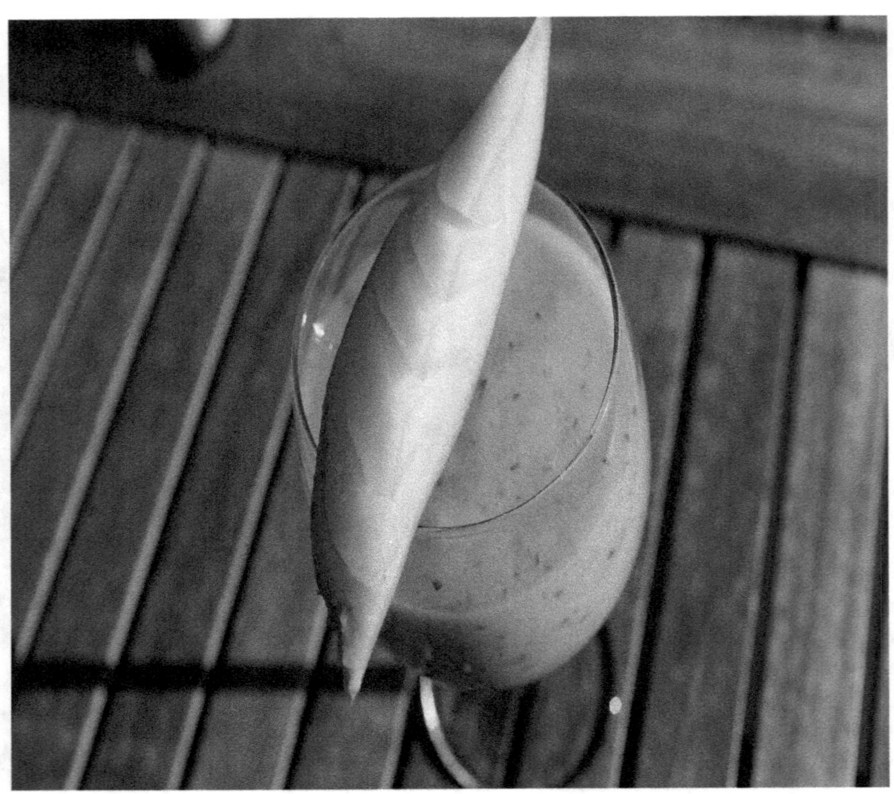

Ingredients:

- 1 cup of mango, sliced
- ½ cup of ice cubes
- ¼ tbsp of honey
- ½ cup of water

Method:

1. In a blender, add all the ingredients.
2. Blend the mixture thoroughly.
3. Serve.

Tomato & honey smoothie

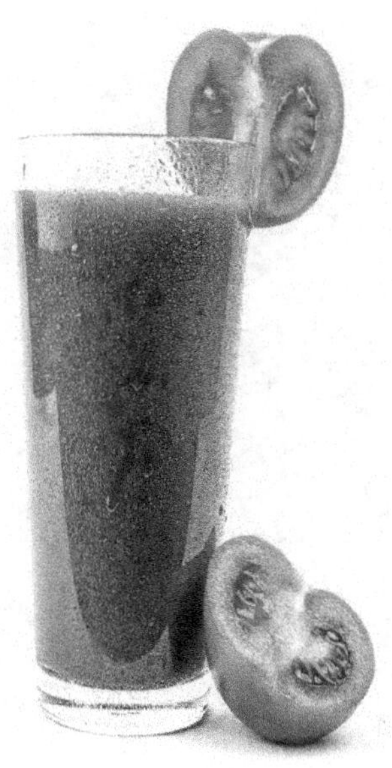

Ingredients:

- 1 cup of tomato, cleaned and sliced
- 1 tbsp of honey
- A pinch of salt

Method:

1. In a blender, add all the ingredients.
2. Blend the mixture thoroughly.
3. Serve chilled.

Raspberry smoothie

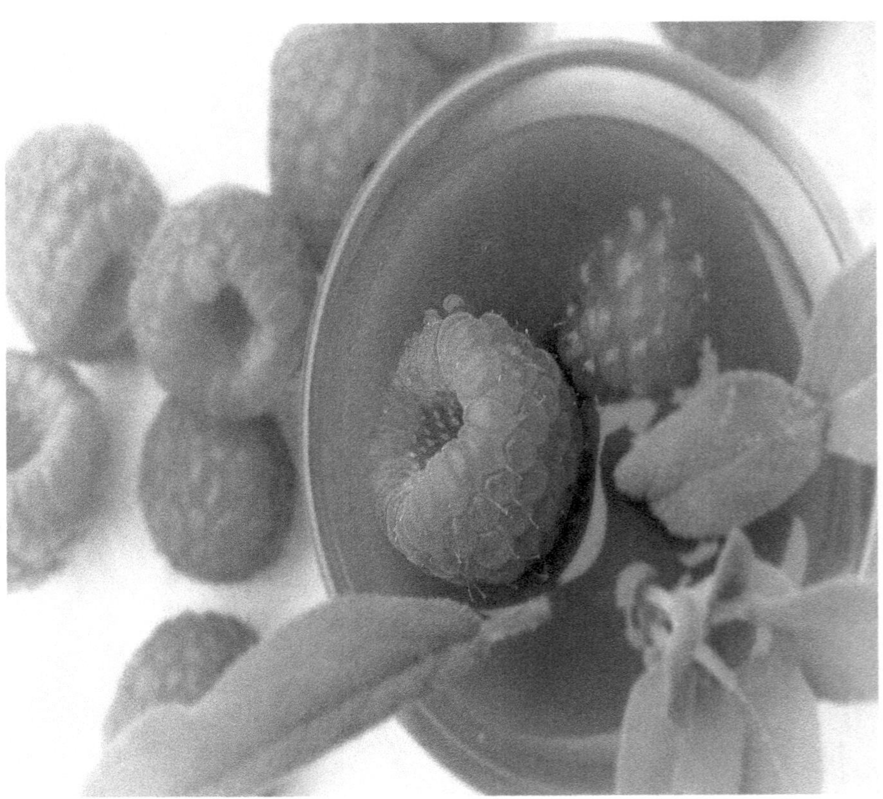

Ingredients:

- 1 cup of raspberry, cleaned
- ½ cup of ice cubes
- ½ cup of water

Method:

1. In a blender, add all the ingredients.
2. Blend the mixture thoroughly.
3. Serve chilled.

Blueberry & banana smoothie

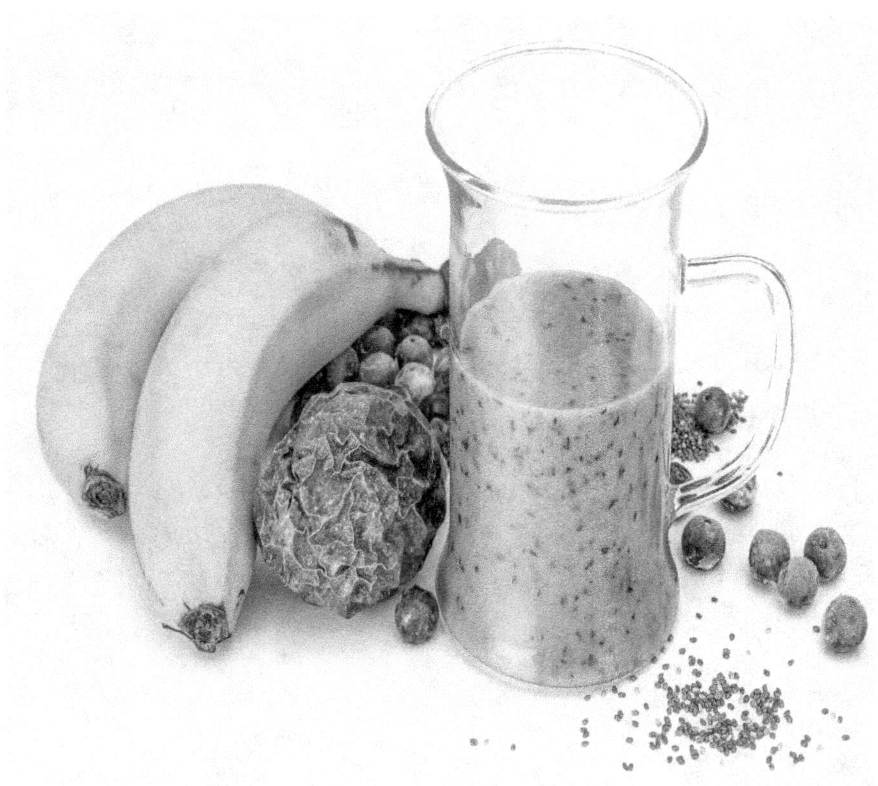

Ingredients:

- 1 cup of blueberry, cleaned
- 2 medium banana, sliced
- A pinch of nutmeg powder

Method:

1. In a blender, add all the ingredients.
2. Blend the mixture thoroughly.
3. Serve chilled.

Strawberry with greens smoothie

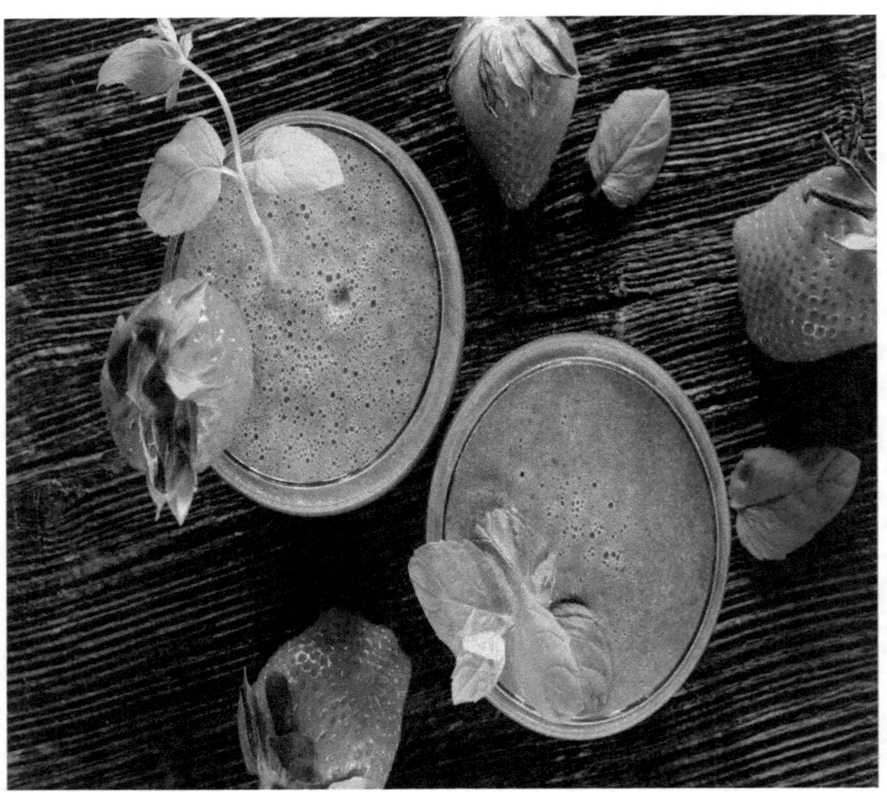

Ingredients:

- 1 cup of kale, cleaned
- 2 tbsp of mint leaves, chopped
- ½ cup of strawberry, cleaned
- ½ cup of water

Method:

- In a blender, add all the ingredients.
- Blend the mixture thoroughly.
- Serve chilled.

Carrot, lemon & beetroot smoothie

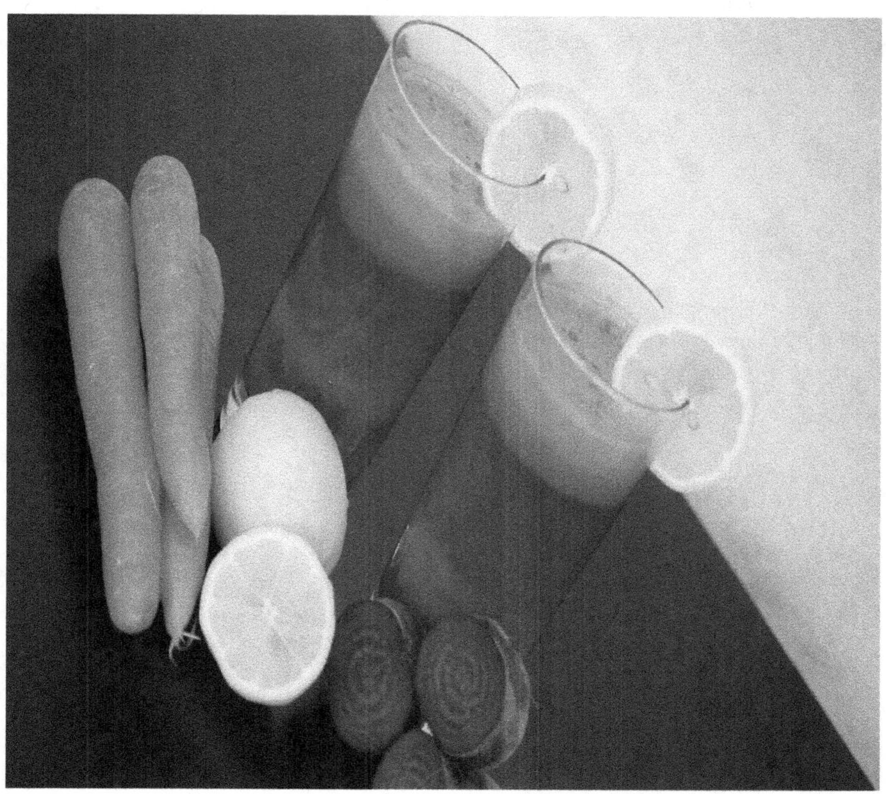

Ingredients:

- 1 cup of carrot, cleaned and sliced
- ½ beetroot, cleaned and sliced
- 1 tbsp of lemon juice
- ½ cup of water

Method:

1. In a blender, add all the ingredients.
2. Blend the mixture thoroughly.
3. Serve chilled.

Mixed berries smoothie

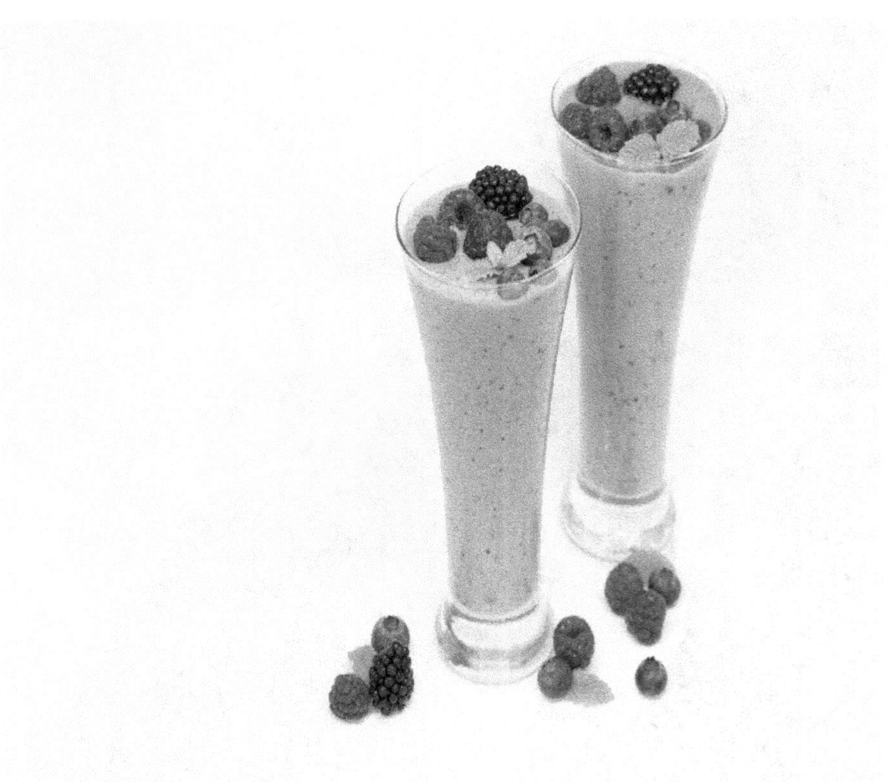

Ingredients:

- 1 cup of mixed berries
- ½ cup of ice cube
- ½ cup of water

Method:

1. In a blender, add all the ingredients.
2. Blend the mixture thoroughly.
3. Serve chilled.

Pineapple & lemon smoothie

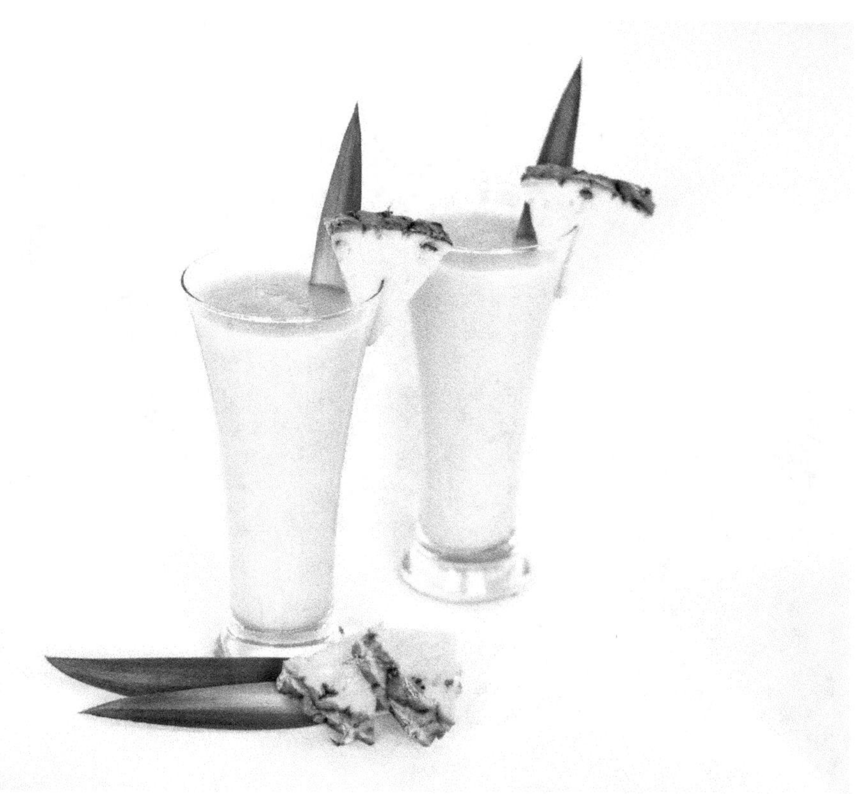

Ingredients:

- 1 cup of pineapple, sliced
- 1 tbsp of lemon juice
- 1 cup of water

Method:

1. In a blender, add all the ingredients.
2. Blend the mixture thoroughly.
3. Serve chilled.

Carrot, beetroot & celery smoothie

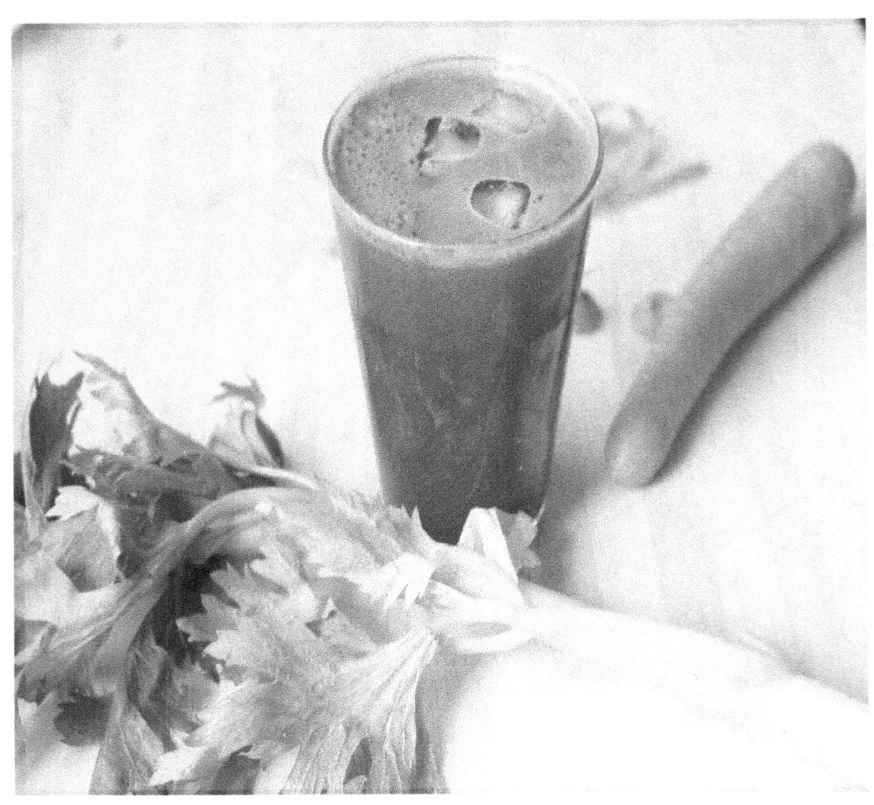

Ingredients:

- 1 beetroot, cleaned and sliced
- 1 carrot, cleaned and sliced
- 1 small piece of celery stem
- ½ cup of water

Method:

1. In a blender, add all the ingredients.
2. Blend the mixture thoroughly.
3. Serve chilled.

Bonus Resources

Thanks for getting this book

Here are some bonus resources that can help you lose weight and keep it off

1. Get Our #1 Recommended Supplement - Exipure

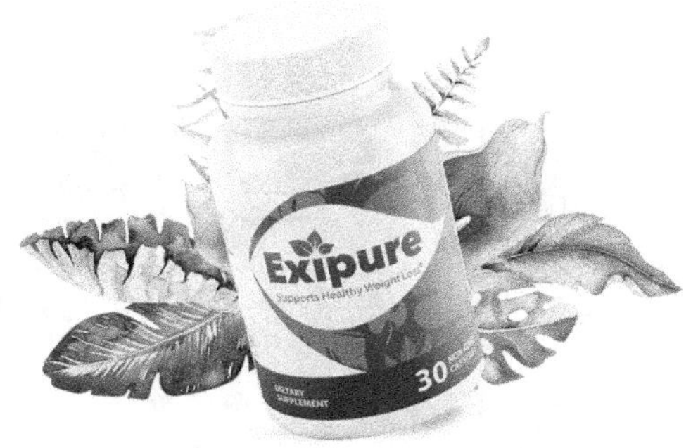

My go-to supplement for healthy weight loss
Get your discount bottle at https://smarterdieter.org/exipure/

2. Join our Recommended Workout
Program - Yoga Burn Challenge

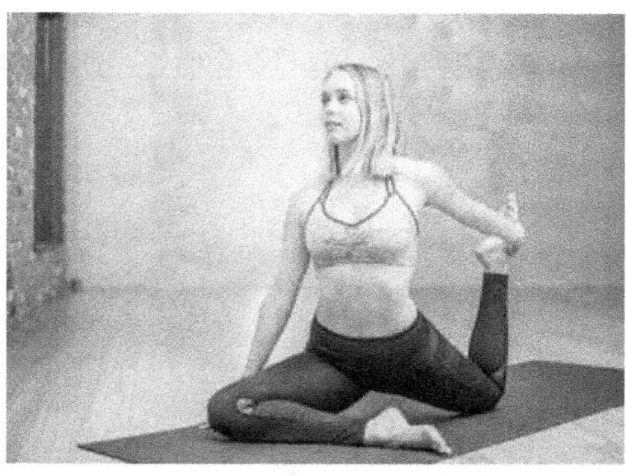

Join the online challenge that will help you lose weight quickly
Sign up now at https://smarterdieter.org/yoga/

3. Join the smoothie diet 21-day weight loss program

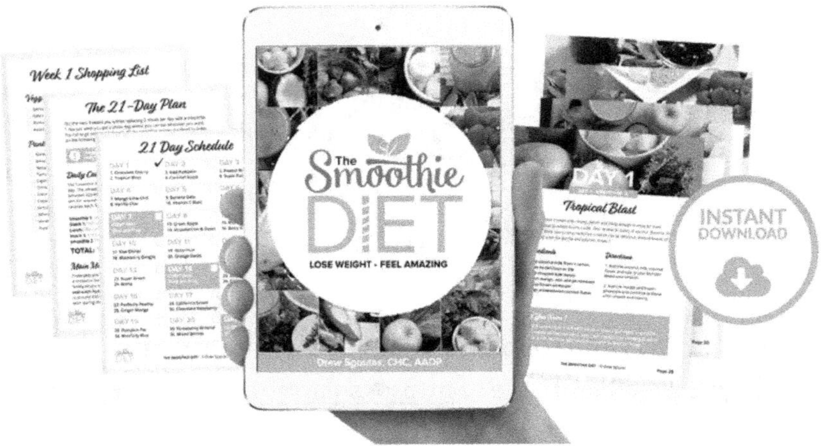

Learn how you can lose weight quickly in just 21 days

Learn more at https://smarterdieter.org/smoothie/